I0414398

Sex & Sensuality

Sex & Sensuality

✦

Essays On Fun Stuff

Nick J. Myers III

iUniverse, Inc.
New York Lincoln Shanghai

Sex & Sensuality
Essays On Fun Stuff

Copyright © 2007 by Nick J. Myers III

All rights reserved. No part of this book may be used or reproduced by any means, graphic, electronic, or mechanical, including photocopying, recording, taping or by any information storage retrieval system without the written permission of the publisher except in the case of brief quotations embodied in critical articles and reviews.

iUniverse books may be ordered through booksellers or by contacting:

iUniverse
2021 Pine Lake Road, Suite 100
Lincoln, NE 68512
www.iuniverse.com
1-800-Authors (1-800-288-4677)

Because of the dynamic nature of the Internet, any Web addresses or links contained in this book may have changed since publication and may no longer be valid.

The views expressed in this work are solely those of the author and do not necessarily reflect the views of the publisher, and the publisher hereby disclaims any responsibility for them.

ISBN: 978-0-595-45985-8 (pbk)
ISBN: 978-0-595-90287-3 (ebk)

Printed in the United States of America

Contents

Acknowledgements

I would like to thank all of my old friends and colleagues from Media Friends School, Strath Haven High School, Old Dominion University, New York University and a select few at Widener University.

I would also like to thank the staff, co-workers, friends and old friends from Settlement Health; the folks at the Family Planning Council—more specifically, the staff from The SafeGuards Project and the Circle of Care. Before I forget, I just want to thank past and former members of the band, Ember.

Finally … just a quick shout out to my old 4-legged friends, Max and Butch. And of course, a very special thanks to Mom and Dad—Love Ya!

Preface

Ok. Let's get this started. Right off the bat, I want to say this book is not important. Well, to be more specific, this book should not be important for you. So ... if you spent your hard earned $11.95 or whatever the actual cost of this book is, all I can really say is that I'm sorry.

You have to understand this is a collection of essays I've written over the past 13 years. This is going to make even less sense when I say I learned how to write after I graduated from college with my undergraduate degree. I was the "set-up" master. Meaning, I would spend the entire document setting up a major point that I would never make or bring to completion.

So, one day I happened to stop by ODU in Virginia and hang out with one of my favorite teachers. She explained to me that I needed information to support my claims. That's all it took for me to make the change but in my opinion, I'm still learning how to write. I've always been the 'idea guy' coming up with great theories and nice concepts but I still have the problem of trying to write them down so the average person can understand my mental processes.

Now, are you starting to get a clearer picture why I said this book is not important? For me, it is a nice time for me to look back and see how far I've come and analyze how far I believe I have to go. In this book, I choose to include one of my favorite essays. In the mid-90's I was a die-hard feminist. Prior to my move to NYC for graduate school at New York University's Program in Human Sexuality, I was reading Mary Daly and Gerd Vandenberg and I was totally enjoying myself so I choose to write an article about female circumcision. I mixed the concepts of physical circumcision through a societal filter where women in American were socialized to 'circumcise' themselves from their body, more specifically their genitals and their sexuality. I called it Social Circumcision: Alive and Well in America. Many of the feminists on campus loved it and told me to publish it. So, I choose to publish it in the SIECUS journal. Well, my article was rejected and, would you believe, in their next published journal, someone else wrote an article on female circumcision in Africa? I was pissed!! What's really funny is that I ended up having an internship in Nassau County, New York with the person who wrote that article. Sorry for the short story but, you must admit that kind of funny. You see, I've written a few articles over the years but I never did anything with them. A few of these are papers I wrote for class at New York University and Widener University. A few I really like while there are others that I'm not too proud of but, I'm going to own them. You mission, if you choose to accept it, is to try and figure out when and where I wrote each article. Ok … I'll give you a hint. More recently, I've discovered my Afro-Americanisms or Negritude. It really opens your eyes when you study to become an expert in your chosen field but you do not see yourself represented anywhere—not in the research, in academia or even in the textbooks (except in the chapter on STDs). Oh … sorry, I was drifting again … Ok … back to this book.

In my attempt to make this book more palatable for those of you who took a chance, I divided the book into a few sections. They are as follows: LGBTQi (I think I covered everyone), Education, African American issues, a few miscellaneous topics and the book ends with a brief epilogue. Ok … now that you're totally confused, I'll explain what each section is made of. Well, here goes!

African-American Issues

When I attended New York University, the main sexuality professor (those of you who know know whom I am speaking of) suggested to me that I explore the sexuality of African-Americans. You see, I was under the assumption that there were bunches of Blacks doing research on the sexuality of African-Americans. Well, I was wrong so, ever since my discovery, I written about the sexuality of African-Americans whenever an opportunity appeared.

One of my favorite essays on the sexuality of African-Americans is Sex: The Black Male's Dilemma. I believe this was my last presentation to SSSS (Society for the Scientific Study of Sexuality) before I was fed up with them. In the essay, I discuss a few variables that have impacted the sexuality of Black males in America. I know I wrote this essay around 1999 and I was pissed off about something but I really do not remember what lit my fuse. For the time being, I will leave well enough alone.

Next, I have an essay called the Black marriage squeeze where I discuss the various variables affecting the low rate of marriage in the Black community. I still find it interesting to talk to professional and educated Black women, of various age groups, about getting married. The women in their early 20's are very optimistic about getting married while the women in their mid-30's are pessimistic about marriage. Many of these women have made the choice to "marry down."

The final essay in this section is a project I did where I had to interview someone about their life. Well, I interviewed 2 interracial couples about their life in American and events that happened to them while traveling abroad. It is an interesting read, to say the least.

LGBTQi

In this section, I have a couple of essays I wrote in the mid-90's while attending NYU. These essays take a look at the lives of LGBTQi individuals in America. I just enjoy reading my old, early opinions about various issues. Don't forget, I said this book in mainly important to me. The first essay takes a quick look at the various ways males in this country are socialized to be homophobic. I discuss a few predictors, or necessary ingredients, to produce a male that has a bias towards gays and lesbians. The next essay takes a more general look at the prevalence of violence and discrimination in gay and lesbian communities. During this period of my life, I thought of myself as being homophobic. I don't know why … I never did anything to anyone; I was never violent towards a person who was gay or lesbians. Now that I look back, I believe I thought I was homophobic because I never knew anyone who was gay or lesbian when I was growing up. Using dumb logic, I felt since everyone else has gay and lesbian friends and I don't have any therefore, I must be homophobic. What makes this logic even dumber is the fact that I had friends and classmate, who I hung out with, who were gay and lesbian! Youth is wasted on the young, isn't it! Finally, the third essay in this section is an essay I wrote in the earlier this decade, probably around 2005. It was on of my last essays about LGBTQi so, I decided to include it in this book. Also, it was well received by a few of my peers so, I tossed it in with the rest. No more … no less.

Sexual Education

Ok … here is the really boring part of the preface where I introduce you to my section on education. Yes, it's very 'textbookie' with very little fun thrown in. That's just how it is. I started this section with a really dry essay about a theoretical model of education. Ok … wait, I know you're aroused and everything but calm down.

The first essay is about the Theory of Reasoned Action (TRA). This education model has been around for decades but I did not discover it until sometime in the late 1990. It's a behavior change model where the person has to believe that they can actually make a change, while having various supports around them. The funny part is that I incorporated this model into a curriculum I was using in NYC. My participants started to use safer sex behaviors but, I was actually using a different model called the Information, Motivation, Behavior Skills Model (IMBS). Oh well … whatever I was doing, it was working.

The next essay is something from around 2002 about abstinence. Believe me, I am and will always be pro-choice. This was an exercise where we had to support an issue we did not necessarily agree with. I guess we were supposed to learn how the other side thinks or look at an issue from a different perspective. I really don't like what I wrote but I put it in this book anyhow. Feel free to skip this one.

This was a tough decision for me but I decided to include 2 essays on sexual dysfunctions. For you, the unfortunate soul who bought this book, there is plenty of information on sexual dysfunctions out there. The dysfunctions I wrote about are dyspareunia and rapid ejaculation.

Dyspareunia is known as painful intercourse. Some women can have pain during and after penile-vaginal intercourse, but it is a mild and manageable pain. For others, it's a totally debilitating pain that requires several days of rest or even medical interventions. A bacterial infection can cause painful intercourse and is easily treatable. For others with no physical symptoms, psychological causes are much more difficult to treat.

The other essay on sexual dysfunctions is a phenomenon known as rapid ejaculation. Definitions vary but it generally understood, if a male ejaculates before he wants to, its rapid ejaculation. But, for some males, they will ejaculate just after penile insertion or prior to insertion into the vagina. Treatments, for the most part, are successful. Learning to know yourself can help you to control your ejaculate. No, I am not trying to minimize the effect of rapid ejaculation on ones self-esteem. All I am saying is that you can train yourself to recognize how aroused you really are. Secondly, if you are a male whose masturbated to orgasm as fast as humanly possible for 15 years, you are going to have to spend sometime un-learning 15 years of behavior.

I also decided to include one of my favorite essays. This is going to sound odd, but I never learned to write in college. I was the 'set-up master.' When I say that, I mean I could spend pages and pages discussing what I was going to talk about and never talk about it.

So, when I finished college in 1994, I was to go to grad school in 1995 so, I started to write. Also, during the period of time, I was a feminist. I used to read Mary Daly all the time. I believe I read 4 of her books including Gyn-ecology, Pure Lust and Beyond God the Father (the last one escapes me now). So, I decided to write an essay on female circumcision. But, I called it Social Circumcision—how females in this country are separated from their clitoris except when sexual pleasure is spoken about in negative terms. I was so proud of that essay and in a way, I still am.

So, I had to go way back in the old, dusty archives to see if I could even find it. Well, it was hidden on an old nasty looking floppy-disk which needed to be defragged before I could even access the files. After all of that, it made it into this unimportant book. (… Funny how I put one of my favorite essays in a book I really don't like that much.)

Miscellaneous

In this last section, I wrote two essays about sexuality that didn't really go anyplace so, I just dumped them here. The first one is about using an internet listserv as an educational tool and the last essay is about swingers.

I think I wrote this essay in 2003. I had just returned to school after a year in Virginia and I was ready to go. Also, I think I wanted to blow the ears off of the professor in my internet class. So, I discussed some of the benefits of using listserv's as a means to get the opinions of a wide range of people on various topics. It was nice and clean at first but I decided to quote a few of the discussions I found/started on a wide range of sexual issues. Oh boy, hold onto your butts!

The last essay in the book is about swingers. The really sad part is that I don't ever remember writing this essay. Don't worry, I'm sure it is mine. It has my 'flavor' all over it and I'm sure it popped out of my brain sometime between 2001 and 2004. In the essay, I discuss some of the various reasons why people join into the swinging lifestyle. Also, I touch on the various types of swingers. Yes, there are different types of swinger—some are way more into the lifestyle than others. Hey … you never know, your neighbors could be swingers. Maybe all of your neighbors swing with each other. That makes the idea of using/borrowing someone's lawnmower seem trivial, don't it?

I decided to end the book with a brief and boring epilogue. For one of my human sexuality classes, we had to write a sexual autobiography. Yes, it a not-too detailed look at my sexual life from the beginning until a few year ago. Trust me, its pretty uneventful. You'll need a cup of coffee just to make it through. But, for you all who decided to read it, I hope you learn something from it. Feel free to compare yourself to my adventures or lack thereof.

Well, thanks for reading my preface. For what it's worth, I wish you well while reading a book that give you a glimpse into my mind over the past decade. Happy Orgasms, NJM3.

1

Sex: A Black Man's Dilemma

Well, you have to admit it is not easy being a Black male these days. White America has no clue what is it like to be 'born a suspect'. Why do guards follow Black males around department stores? Why do people move away from Black males when they enter an elevator? Why do people check for their wallets and pull their purses closer when a Black male approaches? Some of these problems are based on personal fears, which have been supported by the mores of society. If this is the case, has Black manhood been effected by these beliefs?

Black males are now in conflict with the societal definition of manhood. This is a status that a handful of Black males have been able to achieve. Manhood in this society has revolved around a certain level of independence and control over one's environment. In Africa, males knew their status as defined by their society and customs. When they were brought to this country, they were told what their status was and they were given no chance to improve their status. To add, when a Black male did try to improve through education, laws were put in place that made it a crime for him to better himself. Secondly, his status was put in question in the eyes of his family. In many cases, he was unable to maintain a family unit and protect his family from the whims of the slave master.

How are Black males today? This is where things start to fall apart. Black males have to deal with the apparent contradiction between living up the expectations of being a male in this society and the proscription on his behavior and achievement of goals. Therefore, he is subject to the societal disgraces for failing to live up to the standards of manhood on the one hand and being too macho on the other. It is a classic case of "damned if you, damned if you don't". Also, it has been suggested that black males were to effeminate because they were raised in mother-headed households or with a weak father. Currently, Black males are being attacked in literature and at conferences for having adopted a male chauvinist ideal (Staples, 1986).

The social rift between Black males and females begins at an early age. There are internal, external, and societal forces in play here. These forces encourage Black females toward scholastic achievement and discourage Black males from attaining the same goals. Society teaches Black males to prove their manhood through excelling in sports, music, and hustling. In a society that states men are "unacceptable if they are not good looking, professional, with an income of at least $90,000, well-bred, with degrees (p.195), many Black males learn early in life how to gain status in a system that is hostile to them (Chapman,)

It is important to preface, as you read this paper, remind yourself of the concept of internalization. Unless the person takes in a societal belief, it will not be effective. Many of the topics here in this paper have been stewing for hundreds of years. Now, we can see the results in society and in the research. As you read through, ask yourself how things would be different if different 'seeds' were planted years ago.

This papers focuses on five issues that are effecting/affecting the sexuality of Black males in this country. The first issue is emasculation. For hundreds of years, the Black male has had every ounce of his manhood questioned and stripped away. The emasculation began during slavery and has been supported by various reports on the state of Blacks in this country. The second issue is interracial relationships, especially with White women. Why is it that relationships between

Black males and White females causes so much stress? When these two do get together, what are their lives like? The third issue the sexual myths that revolve around Black males. What are they and where did they come from? It is possible the idea for racism was based from the sexual myths of Black males. The fourth issues deals with rape myths. What is a rape myth? Why is it that the research says one thing and society at large still believe another? What are Blacks apparent beliefs regarding rape myths? The final topic deals with sexual dysfunction in Black males. In the final section, you will follow a case study looking at what happens to a Black male when a dysfunction appears.

Emasculation

As the Black male was removed from his African roots, there were extreme changes in his status. During the early times of slavery, black males were encouraged to marry and have children with white women. Only the males from Africa were seen as a commodity. Around 1840 was there an equal number of black female slaves as males slaves. (Franklin, 1939)

After the black females arrived, the black male was forced into the role as the 'breeder' of new slaves for the slave master. The slave master also used the female slaves to gratify their sexual needs. As for the male slave, this is where one of the most important changes in status appeared. During this time, the female slaves' role was more important than the role of the male slave. It was she who raised the children, cleaned the house, and made the food and the clothes. He was put into the role of the females' assistant. It was also common for the mother and her children to be called a 'family' with no mention of the father (Davie, 1949).

The role of the father was gone. To add insult to injury, it was likely the adult male slave was address as 'boy' until he was older when he most likely assumed the title of 'uncle'. Also, if he was married, he was recognized as her husband (e.g. Sally's John) to further lower is status in the household (Elkins, 1963).

After emancipation, the Blacks left the rural areas and headed into the cities where it was hard for black males to find employment. Even though they had skills and were able to work within various trades, they were forced out of these occupations by white workers (Pierre Van Der Berge, 1967). When the black males were unable to find employment, this forced the black female into the role of family provider. The jobs that were available to black males did not have the security nor the income needed to maintain the household. The few jobs that were open to him usually carried the stigma of being women's work (e.g. waiter, cook, teacher, social worker, etc.)(Proshansky, Newton, 1968).

Apart from the history of black males in this country, there have been studies and research used to maintain the ideal of the weak, black male. There are psychological studies that show how black males are de-masculinized, in fact may be latent homosexuals. Their logic is that black males raised in female headed households are more likely to acquire feminine characteristics because there is no consistent adult male model or image to shape their personalities (Pettigrew, 1964). Since black males cannot act in the masculine role, they tend to cultivate female personalities. The result is that the males resemble women who use their personalities to compensate for their inferior status in relation to men (Frazier, 1962).

One of the test that were used to measure the effeminate character of black men is the Minnesota Multiphasic Inventory Test (MMPI), a psychological test that asks the subject the applicability to himself of over 500 simple statements. Black males scored higher on femininity than white males. To prove their point, the researchers stated black men more often agreed with 'feminine' answers such as "I would like to be a singer" and "I think I feel more intensely than most people do". (Hollanson, Calder, 1960)

One of the more infamous writings to appear this century is the Moynihan report. This report had the answers America was looking for regarding why blacks were having a tough time. Yes, the report did mention racism as an important variable but it focused on female-headed households. To summarize the report, it said strong, demanding, independent black women caused the ills that were infecting black males and causing them to fail in American society. The report did talk about slavery and what the slaves had to endure. They focused on how the male slave was emasculated and the result. The next few quotations are from the Moynihan Report and show how the black males were treated:

> "His children could be sold, his marriage was not recognized, his wife could be violated or sold (there was something comic about calling the woman with whom the master permitted him to live a 'wife'), and he could be subject, without redress, to frightful barbarities—there were presumably many sadists among slave owners".
>
> "The slave could not, by law, be taught to read or write; he could not practice any religion without the permission of his master, and could never meet with his fellows, for religious or any other purposes, except in the presence of a white..."
>
> "Negros in bondage, stripped of their African heritage, were placed in a completely dependent role. All of their rewards came, not from individual initiative and enterprise, but from absolute obedience—a situation that severely depresses the need for achievement among all peoples.
>
> "...the slave household often developed a fatherless matrifocal (mother-centered) pattern.

The next sets of quotations are again from the Moynihan Report. These represent the lives of the black male when the report was first published in the late 1960's. They add to the idea of the weak black male and how the black male had acquired the title of 'nuisance' to the household. They are as follows:

> "As a direct result of this high rate of divorce, separation, and desertion, a large percent of Negro families are headed by females".
>
> "Consider the fact that relief investigators or case workers are normally women and deal with the housewife. Already suffering a

loss in prestige and authority in the family because of his failure to be the chief bread winner, the male head of the family feels deeply this obvious transfer of planning for the family's well-being to two women, one of them an outsider. His role is reduced to that of errand boy to and from the relief office".

"The Negro wife in this situation can easily become disgusted with her financially dependent husband, and her rejection of him further alienates the male from family life".

"In essence, the Negro community has been forced into a matri-archal structure which, because it is so out of line with the rest of American society, seriously retards the progress of the group as a whole, and imposes a crushing burden on the Negro male and, in consequence, on a great many Negro women as well."

"Negro husbands have unusually low power."

This shows how scientific research was used to buttress the concept of the 'flawed' Black male. People in this society turn a blind eye to the researcher. They tend to digest the research at face value and take it for what it is worth. Unless another researcher of the same status is able to debunk the research, it stands a good chance of being placed into the mindset of the society at large. Is the myth of the weak Black male still around today? Point taken!

Interracial Relationships

Romantic relationships between Black men and White women have been going on in this country for the past several hundred years. When looking at the history of these relationships, they have been affected by the possibility of beatings, lynchings and death. Less than half a century ago, a Black man could have been killed just for looking at a White woman. Only in 1967 did the Supreme Court declare mis-cegenation laws unconstitutional. When looking at all the marriages that take place, only 1.4% are marriages between interracial couples. Of that number, only .4% are between Black males and White women (Surra, 1991). Today, because of more interactions at work, school, and social groups, there are more chances for interaction between Black men and White women.

Causal Factors

To begin, what causes people of different races to come together and start a relationship? Golden (1959) looked at propinquity as a variable. His research found that people are led into relationship bonds through residential propinquity, economic propinquity, and similarity, both occupational and spatial; by close association and common experiences in the amount, type, and locale of education; and by social contacts.

Number of interracial couples meet on college campuses that are away from home, which reduces the amount of, parental and community control. Robert Staples (1973) felt young people revolted against traditional institutions and values that led them to reject the taboos on dating across racial lines.

Black women usually complain that many professional, accomplished Black men marry unattractive, lower class white women for relationship partners. Merton (1941) felt that such a partner choice represented a "reciprocal compensatory" motivation in which the Black man exchanges his higher economic or professional status for the white woman's higher caste status. More contemporary interracial relationships are more likely to involve partners from the same social class (Pavela, 1964). Furthermore, when a Black woman chooses to enter into an interracial relationship, she will usually choose a partner of higher status than she (Bernard, 1966).

Characteristics

Pavela (1964) concluded from his study that black-white marriages contradict the characteristics of such marriages in the public mind or in the research literature. A few of the following characteristics can be taken from the literature:

> The religiously less devout marry persons of different races with a higher frequency than the religiously more devout (Schnepp, Yui (1955).

Persons who have experienced disorganized and stressful families are more likely to marry members of other races than those who were raised in cohesive and stable families (Hunt, Collier, 1957).

In Black-White marriages, it is the Black male who marries the White female in the majority of cases (Barron, 1946).

Among those who undertake an interracial marriage, a greater-than-average number have been married previously (Golden, 1954)

In Black-White marriages, the family of the Black spouse seems to be more willing to accept the couple than does the family of the white spouse (Golden, 1953).

American male and females marrying out of their racial group are generally older than the average at the time they marry (Golden, 1953).

Consequences

In 1991, for the first time ever, more Americans approved of marriages between Black and Whites than disapproved (Gallup, Newport, 1991). With this being the case, what kinds of problems do those who enter into interracial relationship experience? How do their children develop in the area of personality and interpersonal relationships? What data has been gathered about the consequences of interracial marriage?

To begin, it was found that interracial marriages do not fail less frequently than the average (Lynn, 1953). Pavela (1964) states the idea that the external pressures faced by interracial couples are great but not overwhelming. Some of the larger problems faced by interracial couple are with housing, occupation and, relationships with the family. Many interracial couples are shut out of the social life in Black circles. Therefore, they are forced to seek friends and social contacts in all white or other interracial environments.

The children of interracial relationships appear to be stable. They are considered to be Black by the White and Black community. The children adjust well to the Black community therefore, their problems are the same as those of the children of two Black parents (Risdon, 1954).

When a Black man becomes involved with a White woman, it is likely he will experience some form of hostility and social isolation. Many Black women resent Black men who have entered into an interracial relationship. Those men are perceived as 'selling out' (Pope, 1986). Interestingly, there may be a double standard when Black women date White men. One study asked 350 Black women if they would consider dating a White man? 205 said they had and when asked why, they all said they "want more economic options and a chance at identifying a partner where (they believed) *less hassles would exist*" (Chapman, 1987). {italics mine}

A Black psychiatrist Osmundsen (1965, p.73) said there are "deep seated psychological sickness of various sorts" that underlie most marriages between Blacks and Whites and the participants make use of "the unique opportunity that socially opposed or forbidden interracial sex offers for acting out their personal problems". It has also been said that a Black man who would pursue a White woman purposefully and deliberately to the exclusion of Black woman are exhibiting symptoms of a mental disorder (Akbar, 1979).

Researchers have said a Black man may date and marry a White woman as an act of revenge against White men and a White society that has consistently demeaned him and deprived him of equal rights and opportunity. Whites may view interracial dating as a way to reflect their contempt for the underdog. Some Black men may seize the oppturnity to use a White woman's guilt over racial injustice to negotiate sexual favors (Day, 1974).

Other researchers feel insecurity, self-hatred and a confused racial identity can also be a motive for an interracial relationship. Rejection by peers or by parents may cause an emotional turn to a different racial group. If a Black man seeks out White female companionship, it is said he lacks a crucial aspect of his personal identity that leaves him unclaimed, unsupported, and without the necessary connections with his people and heritage. A White woman cannot give a Black man's life a purpose nor can she share his emotional and historical pain (Pope, 1986).

A Black man is said to suffer in other ways as well. First, possible feeling of anxiety and inadequacy could infect the Black male who experiences feelings of being constantly scrutinized and evaluated by society in general and, by his partners family and associates. Relatives and friends of the white women may prove to be condescending and/or derive some gratification from emphasizing his 'differentness'. The typical concerns with sex roles, dependence, and power will have to be communicated and attended to with a sensitivity to the biracial dimension (Pope, 1986).

Sex Myths

Of all the different races and cultures, it is the black male who has suffered the most because of the white concept of his hypersexuality. Between 1884 and 1900, more than 2,500 black men were lynched. It has been said the black male has a larger penis, a greater sexual capacity and an insatiable sexual appetite. These stereotypes depicted the black male as a primitive sexual beast without the white male's love for home and family (Staples, 1982).

One of the more popular sexual myths deals with the size of the Black male genitals. Black males are thought to have an oversized penis (Fanon, 1967, McCary, 1967). According to the Kinsey Institute, the majority of both White and Black penises measured in their sample were less than or equal to four and a half inches in the flaccid state and less than or equal to seven inches in the erect state (Bell, 1968). However, three times as many Black males had penises larger than seven inches in length. Masters and Johnson reported no additional satisfaction for the female except that caused by the psychological state of the female (Masters, Johnson, 1966).

Hoch (1979) traced the racist theme of the black beast, white hero, and white goddess through the current literature and mythology as far back as ancient Greece. He mentions the perceived menace to the chaste White lady by the ever-erect Black buck has dominated mythology for more than three centuries. Further written accounts of Whites' obsession with Black genitalia and sexual abilities date back to the 16th century. As early as 1550, African religion, skin color and behavior were perceived as being inferior to that of the White Americans (Vontress, 1968). One author linked racism and sexism and examined the means by which depiction of the Black man's sexuality as bestial justifies his oppression (Dworkin 1989). Hoch (1979) speculates the sexual stigma that surrounds the Black males is actually the unreleased, bestial sexuality of white males.

When the Europeans first began to explore Africa, the Africans were defined as pagans due to their religious practices. They were also called savages because of their behavior and they were also thought to have a severe sunburn due to their skin color. The African males were said to have large penises. In 1623, Richard Jobson stated that the Black males were "furnisht with such members as after a sort bothersome unto them" (Jordan, 1968). To restate, the African were inferior to the Europeans in every way except for one—their penis size.

Within the tribal community, their social structure and environment formed values on sexuality. Public rituals often existed to shape improper sexual behavior into a more socially accepted behavior. Whereas Europeans saw sex as inherently sinful, the African code was that sexual breaches of tribal law are offenses against individuals and their social system, not against god (Staples, 1978).

It is possible because of these early interactions; the idea of Europeans being superior to Africans was born. The Europeans defined the Africans as being more animalistic, more primal than they are. They viewed the Africans as being less cultured, less modern than they were. This is where they believed since the Africans are closer to animals than us, we are superior and have the right to control them. Herton (1965) suggests that the sexual stereotype of Blacks may be the single most important factor in maintaining racism.

Rape Myths

There are ideas and concepts in this society that revolve around the causes and possible consequences of forced sexual conduct. Many of these ideas are based on misinformation. This misinformation was given the label of a rape myth. A rape myth was defined as a "prejudical, stereotyped, or false belief about rape, rape victims, and rapists" (Burt, 1980, p.217).

There are several rape myths that abound in this society. For example, the myths include (a) healthy women cannot be raped against their will; (b) women often falsely accuse men of rape; (c) rape is an enjoyable experience for the victim; (d) rape is primarily a sex crime committed by sex-crazed maniacs; (e) rape is an impulsive, unplanned act; and (f) only bad girls get raped (Groth, 1979; Hursh, 1997; McCaghy, 1980; Schrink & Lebeau, 1984; Schwendinger & schwendinger, 1974).

One of the major myths is the typical rape involves a Black male rapists assaulting a White female victim (Epistein & Langenbahn, 1994). It is believed the origin of this myth can be traced back to the days of slavery when the rape of a Black female slave by her White owner was ignored or condoned. But, if a Black male was having sex with White women, even if it was consensual, the Black male was often severely punished or killed. The history books are full of instances where Black males were lynched for having sexual relations with White women. In many circumstances, not only where the males lynched, they were castrated. Hernton (1965) to be a direct attack on the sexual potency of Black males interpreted this lynching-castration by Whites because of the fear of Black sexuality. There was the infamous case of Emmet Till, a Black male who was killed for looking at a White woman (Staples, 1971). In one form or another, some of those beliefs still remain.

Black males who have been accused of rape will usually receive severe punishments (Wriggens, 1983). 50% of those convicted for rape in the South were White males, over 90% of those who were executed for this crime in that region were Black. It is important to note that most of their alleged victims were white. As it stands now, no White male has even been executed for raping a Black woman (Bowers, 1974). But, according to research, 93% of rape cases involve people of the same race (Hirsh, 1981).

The myth of the Black rapist and the White victim influences reactions to rape. Wyatt (1992) found that White women who report being raped by black man was believed more often than those do with White assailants. To add, when a Black women reports she was raped, she is less likely to be believed than White women regardless of the assailant's race.

There are two reports that give some interesting results. Varelas and Foley (1998) conducted a study looking at Blacks and Whites perception of interracial and intraracial date rape. To summarize, this study found if the perpetrator was Black, the participants reacted more negatively than if the perpetrator was a White man. They also attributed more responsibility to the perpetrator and less to the victim. When they looked at the attributions of responsibility of the victim, they found that the White respondents attributed less responsibility to a White woman raped by a Black man that to a Black woman raped by a Black man. In their study, they say, "this reaction may reflect vestiges of the stereotype of the Black male rapist and White victim among the white respondents in the present study" (p. 398).

To add, the Black participants attributed the most responsibility to the Black woman raped by a White man, much more if she was raped by a Black man. This data adds to the idea of Black women not being believed if they report being raped (Wyatt, 1992).

One interesting result of the Varelas and Foley (1998) study found was that the Black participants were more lenient toward the white rapist than toward the Black rapist. The Black participants were even more lenient than the White participants toward the White rapist. When the rapist was White, the Black participants were also more likely to think the victim was responsible and her actions contributed to the rape. The authors said "these reactions indicate that the Black respondents believed in the myth of the Black rapist more than the White respondent did" (p.399).

In another study by Giacopassi and Dull (1986), they were interested in looking at the gender and racial differences in the acceptance of rape myths within college populations. One section of their research focused on racial groupings in relation to accepting and rejecting individual rape myths. They found that only a few of the respondents subscribed to the various rape myths and stereotypes. But, of the respondents who did subscribe to the myths, it was the black males who had the highest percentage of support for the myths and stereotypes. They are as follows:

> The victims of rape are usually a little to blame for the crime.
> A female cannot be forced to have intercourse against her will.
> Rape is usually an unplanned, impulsive act.
> Women often falsely accuse men of rape
> Many females have fantasy dreams about rape (Giocopassi, Dull, 1986).

One should wonder what this research, taken as a whole, really says. In the research by Varelas and Foley, they conclude the Black males actual believe in the myth of the Black male rapist. The research lists what rape myths Black males subscribe to. This is another example of where internalization, the author feels, comes into play. Growing up in a society where one is exposed to this type of 'learning', it only makes sense Black males believe the rape myths. It is almost like, if they did not feel that way, something must be wrong with them.

Sexual Dysfunction

What happens when a Sexual Dysfunction appears in Black males who have internalized the sexual myths? A case study by Wyatt, Strayer and Lobitz (1976) may shed light on this issue.

> Sarah and Nick (pseudonyms) were middle class Afro-Americans in their early thirties who sought treatment at the Sexual Dysfunction Clinic, NPI, UCLA. Nick was experiencing premature ejaculations, which restricted his ability to bring Sarah to orgasm through intercourse, resulting in frustration for both of them. The couple was having intercourse slightly less than once a week with both partners describing their sexual relationship as

"extremely unsatisfactory." Approximately 75% of the time, Nick had difficulty maintaining an erection prior to intercourse. His latency to ejaculation was reported to be less than one minute worth only minimal foreplay.

Sexual Histories: Sarah had been raised in a predominantly black community in another state. At an early age, she became aware of the sexual mores, expectations and stereotypes of her culture, especially the myths regarding black male and female roles. She had been previously married and had a child, age 8. Prior to meeting Nick, she experienced no sexual problems in the marriage or any other relationship in which she was involved. Based upon her past experiences and background, she maintained high expectations of spontaneous sexual relationships, where both partners could perform genital intercourse with mutual orgasm without prolonged foreplay.

Nick's father was a career army enlistee; consequently, Nick was raised and educated in a predominantly white area surrounding army bases where his early social contacts and dating experiences were minimal. His first sexual encounters took place while in the armed forces in Germany. Nick was reluctant to admit a prior history of premature ejaculations because *he was quite conscious of the stereotyped image of the hypersexual abilities of black males. He finally revealed that he felt inadequate that he 'couldn't do his job" of performing up to the stereotyped expectations for his culture.* This performance anxiety served only to heighten Nick's sexual dysfunction. [Italics mine]

In dealing with this couple's problems, there were a few sexual stereotypes they would have to deal with in order to deal with this sexual issue. Most of the more popular sexual myths are reflected here, in both, Sarah and Nick.

Myth: "Black males are naturally sensual lovers".

Example: Nick felt inadequate and inferior because his body build and sexual performance did not "naturally" match the hypersexual black image. His resulting anxiety inhibited him from experiencing physical pleasure during sexual relations.

Myth: "Black women can only be satisfied through intercourse".

Example: Sarah perceived herself as a highly sensual individual who had an increasing need for sexual satisfaction through intercourse. This placed a great deal of performance pressure on Nick. In spite of her self-image, she was not aware of her body's response to physical stimulation other than genital intercourse.

Myth: "Black men and women do not require sexual foreplay before intercourse."

Example: Sarah perceived spontaneous, immediate intercourse as the 'ideal' form of sexual expression. Her early learning history included sexual mores, which proscribed sexual contact other than intercourse

Myth: "Black men have unusually long latencies to ejaculation".

Example: Prior to treatment. Nick denied that he had prematurely ejaculated, attempted to demonstrate longer retention abilities than he had, and refused to admit that there was a history of the dysfunction.

Myth: "All black males are sexually aggressive and highly physical partners".

Example: Nick failed to be as sexually demonstrative and aggressive, as Sarah desired.

Now, here is where we try to sum these ideas into one common theme. This is where one has to go back to the idea of internalization. If the person does not take in concepts and ideas, they will not become a part of the person's mindset and personality. If a person is able to keep from having ideas and concepts become a part of them, they stand the risk of being viewed a different or deviant from the societal norms. Right now, as this is being written, one of the more common ideals regarding Black males is that they are all from the inner city and desire to become rap stars or drug dealers. This image is prevalent on mediums like MTV, BET and several of the more popular television programs. When was the last time you saw a Black male role model who was not connected to the sports or entertainment industry? This is sad to say but a Black male who graduates from college is viewed as atypical. He has done something successful totally outside of the mainstream role he was projected into. Now, return the idea of internalization back onto the five topics covered here.

Emasculation. There is the idea that the Black male has become emasculated because he has been unable to live up to the expectations set by others. In turn, it was the 'others' who set the emasculation wheel in motion hundreds of years ago with slavery. In this century, research was conducted to support the ideal of the emasculated Black male. Think about it. During the times of slavery, if a Black male tried to have something that resembled a household, it would be taken away from him. His 'wife' and children could be sold or killed at the whims of the slave owner. Secondly, if a Black male tried to protect his partner, chances are he would be beaten severely and/or put to death. It was easy for him to see the fact that the slave owner's wife was protected up the house, preserved and safe, just like the angel she was made out to be. Third, the Black male slave also treated his 'wife' as his slave. She was one who was mainly responsible for raising the children and preparing the food (if they had the luxury of food). This is where the concept of the 'no good' Black male began. This is where he would have been viewed as a liability to the "household". The slave owners perpetuated this by the male slave being identified by the females name e.g. Sallly's John. At this point, he had already lost who he was. He was a shell with nothing of his own, not even his own name.

Now, moving ahead to the 20th century, some of the literature supported the idea of the emasculated male. In the Moynihan report, he again blames the Black females for emasculating the Black males. This is where I disagree. At every instance where Black males had the chance to improve themselves, something appeared in the way. For example, after the end of slavery, many Blacks were skilled in various trades. They were ready to work and make something for themselves but were unable to due to the hiring practices of the factory owners. They preferred to hire immigrants from Europe and turn their back to the Black males. So, Black males had to work were they could and just do enough to survive, not live, just survive. They were still empty shells. Only a few were able to make enough and pass it on to their children so they would have something to build on. The others were unable to live up to the standard set by White males and their families. They kept hearing they were worthless and useless so, they actually started to believe it. They internalized those messages. These Black males felt they had failed so, they just existed. Then, these reports appeared interestingly enough around the time of the Civil Rights Movement. This movement was something Black males could get involved in and there were powerful Black males at the helm. They were killed but he was a role model for this generation of men. Now, this report appears to remind Black males they are weak and this time, it is the Black female's fault.

Interracial Relationships. These relationships are nothing new to this country but it is only when a Black male is with a White female that people react. People stop and stare like it is a sin. Actually, some racists quote passages from the Bible saying these relationships should not be. Could these hostile feelings be vestiges from the days of slavery?

During the days of slavery, the White woman was put on a pedestal saying she was to remain pure, unlike the Black female slaves who were viewed as sex incarnate. There are accounts of the slave owners raping the Black females and having offspring with the slaves. There are also accounts of the master's wife blaming the slave for being raped. But, there are instances where the wife would visit the male slaves and have sexual relations with them. Also, it is important to remember before Black female were brought over, the Black males slaves were having offspring with White Europeans to produce new slaves. After this practice ended, laws appeared stating it was illegal for Blacks and Whites to marry. Could it be White America feels Black males are contaminating their White females with their Blackness?

Now, there are two major reasons interracial relationships are looked down on. First, there is the jealously factor projected from some white males. If they see a White woman with a Black man, they become insecure and say 'why didn't she choose me over him'? What they fail to understand is that 1) she was not attracted to you; 2) maybe they have things in common; 3) she likes males with darker skin all year round and 4) she believes the sexual myths about Black males. Second, the bigger issue today is the low number of Black males. Remember, about 1 in 4 Black males are in prison or on parole. Add to that the high death rate and drug about in the Black community [all symptoms of negative internalization]. So, who is going to love the Black females? There is another split forming between Black males and females. Black females today are heading toward higher education and careers. They would like to meet someone who is their equal not someone who will be a liability. There are so few 'good' Black males out there, women are fighting over the men and in some circumstances allowing them to have relationships with other women. Some women just want a male of some form in their lives. As I write this, I have to ask myself what is the definition of a 'good' Black male? My question is was the definition created by Blacks or someone else saying what a 'good' Black male is?

Sex Myths. It only makes sense that the early Europeans used sexuality as a way to demonize Africans. To them, sexuality was connected to the church and god. When they first saw the African tribal behaviors, they were astounded. I am sure some of the African women walked around nude or partially clothed and that was flabbergasting to the Europeans. The Europeans already had stigmas attached to various body parts where the Africans did not. To add, some of the tribal ceremonies were elaborate which included acts of simulated sex. Instead of them trying to learn and understand, their defense mechanisms turned on. This was too much for the Europeans to handle and therefore, they developed the idea that the Africans were closer to animals and therefore should be treated as such.

There is the prevailing myth regarding the sexual stamina of Afro-Americans. For the males, he is always erect, ready at the drop of a hat and can go all night. The sex will be pretty aggressive, hot and sweaty. For the females, she is the seducer, looking for any man to try and satisfy her unquenchable desire for intercourse. Obviously, Whites created these myths. Now, let's spin this around. Is it possible, in these myths, Whites are revealing their own insecurities in the area of sex? Does their own idea of Black sex really threaten them that much? It is possible these myths represent their own repressed sexual desire. These myths are really how Whites would like to have their sexuality but, due to their own stigmas, they are unable to allow themselves the chance for total self-expression. In the Victorian ages, the legs of tables were covered because they were viewed as being sexually exciting. Now, take it a step further after the interracial marriages were outlawed. What was it really that threatened Whites males so much they would pass legislation prohibiting these marriages? Could it be that they did not want Black males 'doing things' to White women they were incapable of? What was said was that Black males were dumb, stupid and undeserving of White women. I feel the actual reason for these laws were based on White male's sexual insecurity. You know the saying…"once you go Black, you never go back!" Well, that saying had to get started someplace.

Rape Myths. These myths go hand in hand with the consequences of interracial relationships. Black male desire to rape White women because they are the untouchables in this society. Black males are dirty and White women are chaste and pure. This is one of the more powerful myths in this society. By way of television programs and other forms of Media, this myth is everlasting.

On various television programs, you see the White women being attacked by a Black male who leaps out from behind the bushes. Then, there is a trial and the male goes to prison. Justice is done, right? Actually, for the most part when a rape is committed, it is against someone of the same race. Research as been saying this for years but the only people who seem not to be listening are in Hollywood.

What they do not understand is that they are feeding this myth. It is telling society the only thing Black males live for is to attack and rape White women. Remember, these people have internalized the same myths that Black males have. They were raised in the same society as Blacks and learned the same myths and messages. I see three main roles for Blacks in Hollywood. They are 1) criminals/suspects, 2) comics or 3) doctors. Rarely are Black portrayed as being regular people. There is always a catch.

Also, notice when a Black male does attack a White woman, it somehow ends up on the evening news. If Nicole Brown-Simpson was Black, do you think the trial would have been such a national phenomenon? On the news, you rarely hear when a Black male does something positive except for when he wins the game by performing a miracle at the last second. When male Black suspects are put in front of the news camera, the viewers get a chance to say 'see…I told you so'.

One important side effect of these rape myths is if a Black male is a suspect of raping a White women, he is guilty until proven innocent. They do not have to show his face in the evening news but they do. It has been shown in the court of law, they believe her word over his. This society has internalized these myths to a point they people are ready to convict him without all the evidence. Researchers who also live in this society did some of the research regarding these myths.

As you read earlier, there was a study that found that Black males believed a list of beliefs regarding rape. Why was this study done? It revealed a population of Black males felt a certain way regarding rape. Then, the research was published. To me, that research looks like it was published to support the rape myths of this society. This research falls again under the 'see…I told you so' banner. People in this society are led to believe all research is done with benign intentions. What this research did was to take the opinions of a few and project them on to all. This is another way to perpetuate the myths regarding Black males and White women. When research like this is conducted, people need to do a Double Think. People need to ask themselves 1) what exact population does this relate to and 2) why was this research really done?

Sexual Dysfunction. This is another example of internalization. The sex myths that are out there have implanted themselves in the mindset of the Black males in this society. Yes, sexual problems are serious but I feel when a sexual problem appears in a Black male, they are far worse for them compared to a White male. Black males now believe if they do not live up to a certain stereotype, they are not men. Their manhood is ultimately challenged. The rules are different for White males. Yes, their manhood is challenged as well as the Black males but, they have the oppturnity to prove their manhood in other ways black males do not. He may be in a position of power at work, be the leader of the household and be respected in the community. Black males also hold this type of status but there is a definite bias. The majority of Black males do not have this type of status therefore, their outlets for displaying their manhood are limited.

If a Black male does have a sexual dysfunction, the problems could be intense. He knows what society thinks of his sexuality and all the baggage that comes with it. The idea of a human sex machine is a powerful curse to live up to. Black males are recognized for their sexual prowess first and their humanity second. The problem is that not everyone can live up to the stereotype. Even the Black males, who choose to 'pass' and live as another race, they cannot escape. You know how society says you are but you know how you really are. Again, you are a failure but this time, you are saying it to yourself. That hurts even more if someone else has said it about you.

For the man above, he had to 1) recognize the myths and 2) that he had internalized the myths so that they were affecting/effecting his sexual behavior. These myths were not read to him so he could memorize them. They were placed everywhere around him so he would ingest them over time so they would be more effective. He noticed how the white parents and children would react to him, how strangers would treat him. He also learned how to grow up by watching the other Black males who were friends of his father. He learned by imitation. Men behave this way and so will I. He watched how White and Blacks would interact. He [read: *we*] are products of our environment. The best way to leave this section would be to state the fact that stereotype can be learned over time but they can be unlearned as well. For this type of internalization, there are no quick fixes.

In the above case study, you have a Black male has a sexual problem. He is suffering from premature ejaculation. He knew the stereotypical requirement to be a successful Black male in the bedroom. When he was unable to live up to the stereotypes, he was no longer a male. He was not a part of the group any longer. Also, his partner had also internalized the expected sexual behaviors of him. So, in this sense, it was a two-pronged attack. He could not live up to the stereotype and he could not satisfy his partner. In this case, the sexual therapy had to reteach [unlearn] this couple regarding their own sexual attitudes and behaviors. This couple was strong enough to risk breaking away from the stereotypes and start seeing each other through clear eyes.

To end this paper, I will start with the question what can be done to liberate Black males from these problems? First, I will say that it may be necessary to throw out the society we have today and start over new. These feeling and myths toward Black males have gone on for so long, they are permanently imbedded in the culture of this country. Sometime we have to be reminded this country was built on death and oppression. If you question this, just ask the Native Americans. In order for this to happen, people will have to give up some of their power and I do not think people will go along with this. I do realize it is wishful thinking to ask for a 'mental revolution' so, we must work with what we have.

Secondly, Staples (1971) believes alternative forms of role fulfillment should be addressed. Because of, employment or underemployment, the Black male will often resort to the virility cult because it is the only outlet he has for a positive self-image and prestige with his peer group. In this industrialized society, we have the means to provide Black males with meaningful employment.

Third, sex education should begin in school as early as kindergarten. These classes should go deeper in sexuality than just the physiological aspects. Males should be taught about the responsibility of becoming sexually active and procreation (Staples, 1971).

Fourth, between men and women, sex should not be used as instrument of domination but as means of communication. The time for game playing is over. Men and women need to cultivate ways of healthy sexual expression which will preserve their basic integrity and humanity (Staples, 1978).

Fifth, we as Black males need to get out of the mindset that we are weak Black males. By perpetuating the myth of the weak Black male on the consciousness of this society, we are doing ourselves an injustice. It is pretty clear that men like Fredrick Dougless, Dr, Martin Luther King and Malcolm X were not impotent eunuchs (Staples, 1971). It only takes one to stand up and make a difference. There are some who need to pick themselves up by their bootstraps. For the others who have their boots laced, it is time to start kicking!

There is one thing I find very interesting. In the movie "Boys in the 'Hood", there is a scene where the father makes the observation about the amount of liquor stores in low-income neighborhoods. I feel they were placed there for a purpose. When you are under the influence of Alcohol, you cannot function well and see life through a fermented haze. You cannot live up to your full potential. Imagine how powerful communities would be if people were able to focus and really see what is going on. Just something for you to think about. Thank you.

2

The Black Marriage Squeeze

This paper is about Black relationships and Black marriage. The author hopes to give the reader a peek into a cultural they may not know nor be a part of. To begin, they are many Black relationships/ marriages that are happy and fulfilling. But, do to a severe gender imbalance, troubling employment rates and early socialization, there are problems in Black relationships. This paper intent is to shed light on a few variables that play a major role in shaping the 'relationship playing field' for Blacks.

In America, the rate of singleness has increased for all, but it is the Black Americans who are the least likely to be married (Bennett, Bloom, & Craig, 1989). They are, as a group, the least likely to get married (Cherlin, 1992). According to the numbers, approximately sixty percent of all African Americans are single (U.S. Bureau of the Census, 1996). It has also been reported that two-thirds of Black marriages end in divorce (Cherlin, 1992; U.S. Bureau of the Census, 1994). Even after the marriage ends, Blacks remain single where other groups are likely to remarry (Sweet & Bumpass, 1987). What is interesting is that most Blacks express a desire to be in a romantic relationship, a significant number will spend a large percentage of the lives being single (Tucker & Taylor, 1996).

A number of studies have shown the decline in marriage rates over the past 40 years. These same studies have also shown the decline in the marriage rates of Black has been greater than the decline for whites. From 1970 to 1990, the percentage of never married Black women increased from 44% in 1970 to 78% in 1990 (Cherlin, 1992).

It is still not known why Blacks have such a high rate of divorce. Some research as found that Blacks report more marital difficulties and less satisfaction with their marital relationships (Chadiha, 1992). This is an important observation because partner satisfaction is believed to be one of the most powerful predictors of an individuals commitment to their partner (Rusbult & Martz, 1995).

Black men and women have the worst gender imbalance experienced by any group since the beginning of the census (Guttentag & Second, 1983). The shortage of Black men in relation to women is largely a function of the high mortality and homicide rates among Black men (U.S. Bureau of the Census, 1991). This variable, added with the high rates of drug addiction (National Institutes of Drug Abuse, 1991), incarceration (U.S. Department of Justice, 1992), and unemployment (Testa & Krogh, 1995) have contributed to a marriage squeeze in the Black community. Because of the low ratio of Black men to women, as many as 25% of Black women in the U.S. many never marry (Cherlin, 1992). I can say I have seen this is my own life. When I walk around campus, I can see the Black women looking at me. Since there is such a shortage, women are really coming after the Black men. I have a few Black women who are just friends and they have already given up on getting married. The sad part is that these women are around my age. They are educated and some are very pleasing to the eye.

Interracial Marriage

One factor rarely mentioned is the impact of interracial marriage. Even though racial endogamy is still the 'rule' for the Black population, marriage rates between Black men and non-Black women are increasing, greatly outnumbering the marriages between Black brides and non-Black grooms.

The intermarriage between Black men and non-Black women may affect the quality of the Black marriage pool by eliminating the most "marriageable" or socioeconomically attractive Black men from the field of eligible mates. These Black men married to non-Black women tend to have relatively high levels of education and occupational prestige. This may affect the marriage prospects of all Black women but is likely to have the greatest impact on highly educated women because intermarriage disproportionately removes higher status men from the marriage pool (Kalmijn, 1993).

I have dated my share of white women. I know the Black women were upset with that. If they found out that I was educated, it was worse. What was really bad was when I used to go to dinner with a white friend of mine. We were just friends out eating a nice dinner and there were a few Black women sitting at a table a few yards away. During the entire meal, every once in a while, they would look over at us. I could not hear what they were saying but their facial expressions were not on the happy side!

Marriageable Men

One of the explanations that has received the most attention is the availability of marriageable men. This theory was based off of Wilson's (1987) idea of the "marriageable male" which says the decline in marriage among Blacks is a result from decreased employment opportunities for Black men. As a consequence of national economic events (read: recessions), unemployment of Black males increased thus decreasing the pool of marriageable men.

History Lesson

Interest in Black male-female relationships developed from the idea that the problems in the Black community came from the inability of Blacks to assimilate into the dominant society. Now, this idea has been named the "Culture of Poverty." This idea states that the social, economic, and political disadvantages shared by Blacks are a clear result of their deviant behaviors and immoral values.

An alternative explanation to the Culture of Poverty idea is the Structural Perspective. This perspective states that Blacks do not have a deviant culture but were placed in a weakened position because of unemployment, underemployment, lack of educational opportunities and other institutional forces that have impacted on their lives. As a result, these conditions caused adaptive behaviors in this community that are considered deviant by the society at large. In order to understand the present, one needs to explore the past. We are our history, correct?

In the early history of Blacks in this country, the Black "family" was forced to live without the stable presence of a father. This was usually do to slavery and the separation of the family by Southern plantation owners. Because of this, the families adapted to this by creating a matriarchal family structure where the Black women were forced to bear the entire responsibility of raising, supporting and socializing the children (Frazier, 1949).

Shortly after the Civil War, legally sanctioned marriages were allowed between the Blacks in an attempt to assimilate former slaves. What was interesting was that marriage between the freed slaves was rare even though the marriages would have been recognized by the state. Because of slavery, the Black women were used to living without the benefit of marriage and being separated from the man who fathered her children. After emancipation, the Black women continued to reject the marital union because it freed her from the subordination of the Black male (Frazier, 1949).

Following Frazier was Patrick Moynihan (1965) with his report called *The Negro family: A Case for National Action*. He felt that urbanization influenced the Black male's ability to financially support his family. Because of this, the Black female took over the role as head of the family. Since there was not a strong male figure in the house, the children were socialized into accepting the Black woman as head of the family. When the Black female children reached adulthood, they did not expect to get married nor did they want to get married for fear of relationship problems coming from the male. The Black male child was socialized into believing his role was to be the biological father of children and leave their raising, socializing and supporting to the mother. This role allowed him to give up his title of head of the family and responsibility for their economic and social well being.

A few years ago, I gave a presentation at a SSSS conference called Sex: A Black's Man Dilemma. I had an entire section devoted to the research and publications that focused on telling how bad the situation was for the Black male. Right here, I could talk about a book called the Bell Curve that pretty much said how Blacks have a lower intelligence than whites. Anyhow, the people who listened to me seemed to understand what I was trying to say. It was well received and the audience asked me several questions {a few of which I was able to answer).

Early Messages

One of the first lessons young Black girls learn is to take responsibility for themselves and their families. The children are taught the skills of survival from the very beginning of life. The values and traditions of the family and culture are transmitted through an oral history, by which the mother passes the traditions and culture down to the children. Black female children are taught that they must be strong and responsible. Black mothers teach their female children that because of unemployment they cannot depend on a Black man to support them and that they must be strong, independent, and economically responsible for the family (Stack, 1974).

At the same time, Franklin (1989) argued while Black women are being taught to rely on themselves, they are also receiving the message of dependency. During their socialization process, Black women hear (a) "Because you will be a Black woman, it is imperative that you learn to take care of yourself, because it is hard to find a Black man who will take care of you," and (b) "your ultimate achievement will occur when you have snared a Black man who will take care of you" (p.216). Even though Black women understand they will be responsible for supporting themselves and their family, the women continue to look for Prince Charming. Disappointment arises when they cannot find a man to support them. The desire to marry and form relationships is there but the reality of life keeps that from happening.

It is generally understood that the socialization of young Black males does not take place with the family but in the broader societal arena, where one encounters traditions of racism and discrimination. This can be explained by referring to Ralph Ellison's book *Invisible Man* (1952). He spoke of a form of 'posturing' exhibited by Black males as a reaction to their invisibility. He felt that racism and discrimination stopped the Black man from showing normal behaviors of masculinity. As a reaction to this, they create symbolically unique postures to combat their sense of feeling invisible. To achieve this, the Black man adopted different patterns of speech, clothing, hairstyles, walking styles and demeanor, all in an attempt to fight against his invisibleness. This was all done to demonstrate to others that he was proud and able to survive against the odds imposed on him by society.

Ellison (1952) observed a posturing that has since been defined as a "coolness" that Black men show as a way to bolster their subordinate position in society and create a positive self-image. Majors and Billson, in their book, Cool Pose: The Dilemmas of Black Manhood in America (1993) felt because of the high unemployment rate, Black men are often unable to fulfill the traditional role of the male as the provider and breadwinner for the family. Because of this, Black men adopt a 'cool pose' as a way of defining and maintaining their masculinity. Black men often become detached and cold, displaying an outward appearance of indifference to the circumstances around them and to the women involved in their lives. These men loose touch with their feelings and the ability to develop/maintain healthy relationships. The persona of "cool" is a coping strategy used my Black men in order to deal with the frustration, rage, and anger coming from the inability to provide for themselves and their family. Many show their manhood through procreation and promiscuity.

In terms of the Black male/female relationship, the 'coolness' creates a barrier between them. Majors and Billson (1993) felt during the initial stages of the relationship, the woman actually seeks out and encourages the 'coolness.' The display of detachment, strength, and sexual prowess is attractive to her. But, after the relationship starts, the very item that attracted her to him prohibits the development of an intimate relationship. Further, when a crisis the male cannot handle appears, he reverts back to the 'coolness', which reinforces the barriers in their relationship.

I have several friends who would fit into that mold. Many times, I fall back into that 'coolness' behavior because I know it is safe. I have to say it is tough to keep the barriers down. Every once in a while, things just get so bad that you have to keep the 'coolness' running 34-hours per day. It keeps people away from you and it creates time where you can begin to center yourself again. But what usually happens is that you don't get enough time to sort things out and the 'coolness' comes back again, sometimes ever stronger.

Commitment

> "... *aside from postwar shortages of men in various countries, American Blacks present us with the most persistent and severest shortage of men in a coherent subculture group that we have been able to discover during the era of modern censuses.*"
>
> —(Guttentag & Second, 1983, p. 199)

Its has been stated that a strong male/female imbalance in any society would cause havoc between the genders. Guttentag and Secord (1983, p. 20) outlined the possible consequences of a significant gender imbalance in cases where there are shortages of men:

> "Women in such societies would have a subjective sense of powerlessness and would feel personally devalued by the society. They

would be more likely to be valued as mere sex objects. Unlike the high sex ratio situations, women would find it difficult to achieve economic mobility through marriage. More men and women would remain single or, if they married, would be more apt to get divorced. Illegitimate births would rise sharply. The divorce rate would be high, but remarriage would be high for men only. The number of single parent families headed by women would increase markedly ... The outstanding characteristics of times when women were in oversupply would be that men would not remain committed to the same woman throughout her childbearing years. The culture would not emphasize love and commitment, and a lower value would be placed on marriage and family. Instead, transient relationships between men and women would become important."

This concept suggests lower commitment to romantic relationships coming from the gender group in shortest supply. Therefore, the existing gender imbalance experienced by Blacks probably reduces romantic commitment of Black males. On the other hand, the lower ratio of Black males to females should reduce the number of alternatives for Black females and increase their level of romantic commitment.

One study found that satisfaction with the relationship and the availability of romantic alternatives were significant predictors of commitment for Black females but only the availability of romantic alternatives was a predictor of commitment for Black males.

The same study also looked at differences between the races. It found, when compared to White males, commitment for Black men did not increase as satisfaction with the relationship increased. It is possible since Black men are in such short supply, they know alternatives are always available to them. Therefore, it is possible that the level of commitment could be decreased with the reasonable expectation that better or equal alternatives are available to them (Davis & Strube, 1993). It is important to remember that Black males are not totally controlled by external factors. They can respond to changes in their values, social pressures, and opportunities. We can assume that

Black males also have a "hedonic calculus" built into their psyche. That is, Black males make the decision to enter, stay or leave their relationship based on their perceptions of its overall benefit to them (Rusbult, Johnson & Morrow, 1986a).

Research revealed that Black women adhered more closely to traditional marriage norms as they place more importance on economic supports in marital timing decisions and are more resistance to marrying a man who has fewer resources or who has had a previous marital/family experience. Black men also report they are open to marrying a woman who has greater resources than they, place more emphasis on economic support and are less willing to marry someone with previous marital/family experience.

Based on the information from the same study, the marriage rates for Black females is most likely declining because of a lack of available Black males who can meet a Black woman's high expectations for male family headship (i.e. greater resources), a recognition by both Black males and females that their economic criteria for when to get married are not being met, and a greater unwillingness to marry someone who was previously married (Bulcroft &Bulcroft, 1993).

I know my standards for picking and staying with a partner are pretty high. I know what she had better look like and the body shape I prefer. She had better had nice legs and a kind of butt that I can grab a hold of. I know they are out there because I see them all of the time. If I see one who interest me, we can talk. If we get together and she starts to get on my nerves, she is gone. No question. I am used to the 'lone wolf' role and I have no problem telling a women who is getting on my nerves to get lost. Since I know the numbers are in my favor, I really do not have any worries.

Staying Together

There was research that looked at marital happiness between dual-career Black couples. There are very few studies that looked that the marital happiness between Black couples. Most of the research published focused on the harmful variables that affect Black relationships.

This research found happiness with ones employment took on additional importance as a determinant of global life happiness. The importance of job life to global happiness seems to have an important correlation. It also found that dual-career couples depend on their marriages for their overall happiness and psychological well being (Thomas, 1990).

The spouses were happy with their lives. It could be that the multiple roles (e.g. spouse, parent, employed person) provided gratification, security, increased self-esteem, and a strong sense of purpose. It has been argued (Thoits, 1983) that multiple roles can be generally beneficial.

Right now, I cannot think of too many Black couples that are from my parent's generation that are still together. I can remember couples from my grandparent's generation who are were together but many of them have passed on. So, I wonder if the problem could be a lack of role models for people in my generation?

When it's Over

One study found of the Black men who had conflict with their relationships said it was only a few variables that were causing the conflicts. They reported irritating personal habits (punctuality, cleanliness, preferences, etc.), how to spend leisure time, being away from home too much, time spent with friends and the job were the major areas of conflict (Gary, 1986).

Among those Black males who experienced considerable conflict with their partner, there was the tendency for them to report a high level of depressive symptoms. Some antisocial or deviant behavior, such as excessive drinking, drug abuse, suicide attempts, and violence which are prevalent in the Black community may be a manifestation of the level of interpersonal conflict with women that many black men are experiencing in their daily lives (Gary & Leashore, 1978; Staples, 1978).

As it was stated earlier, it is not very clear why the divorce rate among Blacks is so high. Some research has shown that Black men and women report more difficulties and less satisfaction with their marital relationships (Chadiha, 1992). It is believed that partner satisfaction is one of the most powerful predictors of ones commitment to their partner (Rusbult & Martz, 1995). This question is does this research hold true for Blacks as well?

One study looked at the way couples would perceive their level of happiness when they were asked to project beyond their current marriage. In general, the study found that Black spouses reported perceiving life outside their existing marriage less negative than their white counterparts. For example, Black wives reported anticipating that their sexual and social lives outside of marriage would be more favorable than staying in the marriage. Black males may feel that, because they are fewer numbers, they are in greater demand. Black women, on the other hand, may feel their chances of finding alternative partners are also good given Black's higher divorce rate and larger pool of never married men. What is really interesting is the same study found that Black husbands and wives perceived that their standard of living would suffer less in the absence of their present spouse (Rank & Davis, 1996).

Most Black women entering into their first marriage will not remain continuously married until either they or their husbands die. What is more likely is, in about 65% of the marriages, is that she will separate from her husband (Martin & Bumpass, 1989). Approximately 45% of the separated Black women will attempt a reconciliation (Wineberg, 1994b).

The chance that reconciliation will be successful varies by 1) the age at separation and 2) whether or not she gave birth before marrying. Women who separate after the age of 23 are more likely to have a successful reconciliation than women separating before age 23. Older women are generally more mature and more disciplined than younger women and it may be easier for them to make the sacrifices necessary to have a successful reconciliation. The younger women may believe as long as they love their husband their marriage can be saved and they may not consider all that goes into making a marriage work. Also the younger women may have less incentive in getting back together since they may have less invested in the marriage than women who are older when they separate (Wineberg, 1996).

Second, women who give birth before marriage are much more likely to have a successful reconciliation. It is believed that it is the timing of the birth that affects the success of reconciliation. It is possible that women who gave birth before marriage may have a strong commitment to the institution of marriage in that they were not forced into marriage by a premarital pregnancy. A couple who highly committed to marriage may exhaust all options to save the marriage and also may tolerate substantial marital discord before deciding to end the marriage (Wineberg, 1996).

To develop programs and policies for improving relationships between the sexes in the Black community, conceptual clarity is needed to define the problem and its causes. Franklin (1980, p.47) stated:

> "The familiar rational offered for Black male-female conflict, white racism, is deemed logically inadequate ... To be sure, not all Black males and females experience undue difficulty in social interactions ... It is suggested that the conflict stems from the diverse manner in which some Black males and females define situation, interpret each other's behaviors, and direct action toward each other."

Through this paper, I have taken the reader through a time capsule. In brief, we went from American slavery up to the present. If you come away with one thing from this paper, it should be that Blacks, as a community have it tough. It is nice to see report on the news about how race relations are getting better between everyone but, you have to take a look inside the cultural to understand what is really going on.

The author must emphasize that not all Black relationship are negative. Not at all. Many are happy and very well adjusted, but you rarely ever hear about them. It seems that the society as a whole enjoys making Black life look dysfunctional. Then, society uses that apparent 'dysfunction' as an excuse to maintain various ingrained social traditions such as racist behaviors and social stigmas. It will be a great day when the research on the Black community actually reveals/reflects the truth.

I would like to add a personal message for all of the researchers out there who are currently doing research on people of color, especially on Blacks. Browning and Miller (1999, p.647) sum up my feelings pretty well. They write:

> "... The cultural of poverty theorists impose their bias and ideology on the lives of the people they studied. When they observed differences, they attributed those differences to a deviant culture pattern. To some extent, bias is inherent in all research. The researcher does not undertake research that is not of interest to him or her. On some level, they have an ideal of the relationships between the variables within the study and the expected outcomes. This could, of course, inform their hypothesis and the way data are interpreted. However, having said this, it is the responsibility of the researchers to recognize their bias and to the best of their ability not incorporate it into their research. It appears that the research conducted by the culturalist was informed by their bias. When faced with the structural reality that Black males were either unemployed or underemployed at a rate higher than white males, the culturalist interpreted the lack of marital unions and the messages passed on to the children within the Black community as the result of the domineering Black woman, not the obvious structural limitations facing the men and women in the community."

◆　　　◆　　　◆

Addendum

Well, I can say I didn't really learn anything new. All of the things I wrote about in this paper I always heard about, lived or observed while I was growing up. Nothing really shocked me. You're probably wondering "… so, why did you write this paper?" Let's just say I wanted/needed some conformation regarding a few issues.

I heard about the idea of the marriage squeeze in the Black community for awhile now. Ever since I can remember, actually. Now, I understand why my small family invested so much in me when I was small. I am a Black male with potential. I can remember when I was sick or something, I didn't go to a doctor, I went to a specialist even though my family could not afford it.

Since I was raised by women, my mother instilled some of the same values in me that my grandmother put in her. I like to say that I modeled myself after my mother in the early 80's. She was a very independent woman who used to kick ass and take names when she felt like it. She raised me to be independent and not to rely on others for help. Then, my grandmother taught me how to "do things." Now, I am a good cook, I can take care of a garden and take care of small problems around the house. All of my friends who were raised by single mothers are just like me. Some are married and the guys are better cooks than their wives are.

You see, the messages I received when I was small to learn how to survive and take care of yourself. People will come and go in your life but you will have to live with yourself for the rest of your life. Those are just a few of the messages I got.

As for the Moynihan report, blaming Black women for the problems of Black men was just plain wrong. {if you haven't read it, you might want to take a peek!} Yes, the Black women I grew up with were strong and are still strong now.

As for the interracial dating/marriages, I have no problem with that. When I was younger, I dated my share of White women. One of my oldest friends on the planet is in an interracial marriage. {She's a nice girl but she can be flaky sometimes, but hey …!} I also know some Black women who get upset/angry/hostile when they see a Black man with a non-Black partner. I think they feel it is smack in the face. The market is tight to begin with so I can understand their hostility.

Personally, I think their anger grows especially if they know that the Black guy is about something (educated, nice job, car, looks good). My mom always tells me about how good I must have it in the dating game. I just tell her I'm not in the mood to play the game.

One of the biggest problems I had in writing this paper had to do with the general bias in the articles. There were so many articles on why/how Black relationships were going to fail, it was overwhelming. There were almost no articles on what makes Black relationships work. I only found a few on successful Black marriages. It was weird but I'm not surprised. I guess, every once in a while, I have to remind myself of why I got into this field. It's such a shame. I guess the researchers were much more interested in proving their own point [agenda] in explaining to society that Blacks are dysfunctional.

Deep down, I guess I knew what I was going to find in the library. The libraries really don't change no matter where you go … the pages still say the same thing. Since I've been in this field, I've always wanted to so some serious work on Black sexuality and try to make it as good as it could be for as many people as I can. I know I have a lot of work to do before I die. See ya!

3

Techniques for Coping with Public Harassment by Interracial Couples

"Does the public harassment bother me? Well, it depends on what day it is. It builds up over time, until you're really sick of it. I can truly say I don't care what other people think—but I don't care to be reminded every ten minutes that I am with a Black man and of the travesty I'm doing to society. In my mind, we are all humans—and if you don't think so, then you are the one with the problem."—A white woman in her twenties engaged to a Black man (Datzman & Gardner, 2000, p.6).

Even though racial intermarriage has been rare, evidence shows that during slavery, sexual contacts between Blacks and whites were not uncommon (Williamson, 1980). Although the "mixing" of Blacks and whites in this period may have occurred, there was a consistent system of extreme racial inequality and strong anti-Black prejudice (van den Berghe, 1967). Because the dominance of the white majority was stable, clearly defined, and heavily protected by institutional arrangements, whites generally had little fear of interacting with Blacks in a more intimate social environment.

When slavery was abolished, a gradual decline in formal inequality of Blacks and whites walked in parallel with the growing anxiety about the social boundaries between the races. When looking back, later researchers noted the increasing attempts by whites to keep the races separate in social arenas (Myrdal, 1944). Myrdal (1994) also mentioned that within the social sphere, anxiety between the races increased when the contact was more intimate. Interracial dating and marriage were condemned and strong social norms emerged against interracial contacts with possible erotic undertones, such as interracial dancing and swimming. Jim Crow laws formalized segregated public facilities and legislation controlled interracial sexual and marital contacts (anti-miscegenation laws). Anti-miscegenation laws were in place both in and outside the South, were the penalties were generally most severe in states with larger Black populations (Wirth & Goldhamer, 1944). Further attempts to separate the races were supported by the creation of the "one-drop—rule," a system of race classification that socially and legally defined all mixed children as Black (Davis, 1991).

In 1967, the Supreme Court declared the laws banning interracial marriages were unconstitutional. Most of these marriages follow a pattern of Black man/white woman partnerships. The idea of racial endogamy and certainly the fear of discrimination and harassment are some of the main deterrents cited for interracial marriage and interracial dating (Zebroski, 1999).

Among other issues, attitudes towards interracial dating vary by race, with white holding more positive attitudes than Blacks, men more positive attitudes than women, and younger people more positive attitudes than older persons (Todd, McKinney, Harris, Chadderton & Small, 1992). Complicated circumstances lead to Black/white interracial relationships, and hypergamy/hypogamy considerations do not explain each couple's decision, at least not in any simple way (Moore, 1999). An important factor in disapproving attitudes is the accusation of status hypergamy toward those who marry whites (Kalmijn, 1993). A Gallup poll found that 66% of U.S. college student say that they approve of interracial dating, while only 7% of them report actually having engaged in interracial dating (USA Today, 1997).

Individuals who noted some of the disadvantages of interracial dating and romance have been know to name the discomfort to which they have been subjected in public places. Others who have discussed their interracial marriage also identify the same circumstance as hurdles to overcome (Mathabane & Mathabane, 1991).

In this research, I am interested in interracial couples' management strategy for dealing with problems created by people they have met in public places. While I am interested to the couple's reactions to the negative experience (shock, numbness, sadness, anger), I am more interested in how they dealt with the situations. Some management strategies could include:

1. Ignoring—Purposefully ignoring or repressing the public harassment.

2. Avoiding—Staying home or attending a private gathering that was guaranteed to be receptive.

3. Presence Alignment—Minimal or silent agreement by partner who witnesses, but does not actively participate in, the other partner's more obvious rejection of the harassment.

4. Segregating—Couple choose to enter places filled with 'their own kind.'

5. Accompaniment—Choosing reinforcement by numbers (aka—'strength in numbers).

6. Answering Back—verbally attacking the individual(s) who are harassing you (Datzman & Gardner, 2000).

In this research, I hope to explore and document the management strategies used by interracial couples for dealing with public harassment. The management strategies used by interracial couples exist because they disempower the harassment, in whatever form the harassment appears. At the same time, the strategies are empowering because they allow the couple to protect themselves from racism (Hill & Thomas, 2000). When looking at the bigger picture, the strategies relate to the heart of America's cultural assumptions about who may or may not be one's romantic partner.

Method

The purpose of this qualitative study was to explore and describe interracial couples' management strategy for dealing with problems (harassment) created by people they have met in public places.

The sample in this study was made of two interracial couples. Both couples were made of a Black male and a white female. Names have been changed to protect the innocent. The first couple, Kevin and Sarah, currently lives in Delaware County. Kevin is 35 and works as an inventory consultant for an international corporation. Sarah is 27 and is a paralegal for a law firm in Philadelphia. They met through Sarah's sister while Kevin was playing in a local band. They are married with a total of 3 children, including one child from a previous relationship involving Sarah.

The second couple, Yngwie and Marti (they made up their fake names), also lives in Delaware Country. Yngwie, the male, is 33 works as a paralegal for a law firm in Philadelphia. He is a singer/songwriter who performs locally. He also has a couple of CD releases to his credit. Marti is 30 years old and is a teacher who works with ESL students who just graduated from the University of Penn with a Masters in education. She is also a singer/songwriter with a CD released. They met at a local spot in Philadelphia called The Lion Fish, which was known to offer acoustic/folk music. She was looking for a place to play while Yngwie was a fairly established musician in that community. They have been a couple for over 3 years and are planning a move to Los Angeles to further their careers.

When I approached my potential interviewees, I was forthcoming due to my reasons for wanting to include them in this study. At the same time, I was reserve in offering the actual focus of the questions. The interviewees were more concerned about my previous education. Since the researcher is known, by all of the interviewees, as being involved in the human sexuality field, some were concerned about the nature of the questions. I assured them that the focus of this study was not on sex and their sexuality. It should be noted that Sarah comment that this researcher had been *"Blacklisted"* due to my academic and career aspirations.

The interviews were taped. The interviews were conducted in their homes. Due to time constraints, this was the most convenient method of gathering data. The interviews lasted between 45 minutes to an hour. No follow-up interviews were necessary. In conducting the interviews, the researcher used a combination of the informal conversational interview and the general interview guide. From the informal method, the researcher supports the idea of spontaneous questions and natural interaction. Since this is more like a conversation, in contrast to a tightly structured interview, the researcher believes this style would put my participants at ease. But, at the same time, there are specific topics that are important to explore within the interviews, which comes from using the general interview approach.

Face-to-face interviews offer a greater chance to obtain an accurate understanding of a person's harassment experience along with their management strategy. It allows for personal contact that may increase the likelihood of an interviewee sharing more information if the researcher offers support and encouragement. Face-to-face interviews also offer more in-depth data. According to the literature, face-to-face interviews are more likely to offer the most complete, accurate, and unbiased information than any other method of data collection (Epstein & Tropodi, 1980).

Results

When reviewing the data, there were some correlations with the strategies listed above, as well as, strategies that were not listed. In this research, the couples reported using management strategies that included ignoring, avoiding, accompaniment and segregation.

Ignoring

One couple spoke about ignoring or repressing public harassment. In other research, 'not reacting' was sometimes savored as the moral high ground; a piece of wisdom that is common in the etiquette system of the U.S. for dealing with bad behaviors of others. The couples that were being harassed felt that their harassers had broken a fundamental norm of 'live-and-let-live'. By not responding, they were not 'descending to the level of their tormentors,' but showing that they were 'better' than or even 'more civilized than' their harassers (Datzman & Gardner, 2000). In this research, Yngwie and Marti commented on laughing off a situation. Initially, Yngwie is talking about how he thinks other people view him because he is dating a white woman but Marti changes the topic:

> *Yngwie*—People tend to think that I think that I'm so good ... hot shit.
> *Marti*—... or, you've got money ... there's money involved.
> *Yngwie*—I haven't noticed a lot of negative reaction.
> *Marti*—Remember when we were first starting out and we would go to Dunkin Donuts and there was that group of old men ... at the table, who would scowl at us? But, I don't know if they were scowling at everybody or just at us.
> *Yngwie*—... I just felt they were old bitter guys.
> *Marti*—Do you remember that drunk guy ... when we were on South St., who was sayin some stuff to us? There was this guy ... I cant remember if it was New York or South Street and he was talking about how ... I cant even remember exactly what he said ... it was some kinda lude comment about ... some kinda Jungle Fever comment. He was obviously drunk and we just kinda laughed it off and the people around us kinda laughed it off.

What is interesting here is that the other people around them also knew of the ignoring social norm. The people around them were able to figure out, with relative ease, who the comment was directed to and respond accordingly. Laughter is a great way to take the power away from a harasser.

As was mentioned earlier, Kevin and Sarah have interracial children. Sarah discussed a time, while at a local McDonalds, she encountered a group of older women. Instead of ignoring the questioning, she actually answered the question, which is an interesting strategy within itself. After she describes the event, she asks an interesting question, which could reveal her insecurities about actually being their mother:

> *Sarah*: What kinda category would they put the kids in? As an example, I went out to breakfast with the kids (the two youngest/ interracial children) and "B" was in school (the oldest child from a pervious relationship; similar skin tone to Sarah). I went to McDonalds. There were like four old people, like white-haired old people sitting at one of the tables. And the kids ate and whatever and we're getting ready to leave ... ya know, 'Come on guys, lets go.' And this one old lady ... and again, she meant well but, it's one of those things were people don't think before they speak. And she goes, 'Excuse me ... did you adopt those children?' And I was like 'No ... they're mine'. Mixed kids look like they could be ... Spanish ya know, or Italian ya know ... I just found out The Rock (from WWE wrestling) is Black. I thought he was Italian.
>
> *Kevin*: If you remember, I was working 6 days a week. So, I rarely went out with them. I never noticed anything. But then again, it's not as obvious in my case when they're out with me. They are *certainly* much darker than you are (said to Sarah).
>
> *Sarah*: The only thing I've noticed is that people think I'm babysitting ... I usually get the 'double-take' look ... but that old lady was the first one that ever just came right out and asked me 'did you adopt them,' you know. *Do they not look like me at all?*

Accompaniment

One strategy discussed by one of the couples was called accompaniment. This could also be known as the strategy that involves 'strength in numbers.' More specifically, the interracial couple chooses rein-forcement by numbers that are known to be supportive. One of the Black males interviewed said:

> *Kevin*—Which is part of the reason ... I don't think I discussed this with you (directed to Sarah), but I'm more comfortable being here because I know enough people who will look out for my family. There are enough people that I know ... (pointing) over there, over there ... ya know, all around ... including police offic-ers too, that will definitely make sure everybody is safe.

Avoiding

Avoidance was another commonly reported strategy used by interra-cial couples for avoiding harassment (Gardner, 1995). People put this strategy into practice by choosing to stay home or attend a private gathering that was guaranteed to be receptive. In doing so, they sought to shield themselves from the unpleasantness or even possible danger of public harassment by screening out those they considered possible harassers. In discussing two distinct sections of the Delaware Valley, Yngwie and Marti commented on their social activities:

> *Yngwie*—I'm not involved in Chester. I live here but I really don't know anyone. I'm not really involved in it so it makes it harder for us to go out for a walk. I mean ... people go out for walks, in Chester, all the time, I'm sure. Women go for walks ... white women go for walks in Chester but, that has nothing to do with it. But, I'm not involved in it and so, I'm more on the defensive in Chester, with us. Partly because of anything racial but that's how I was before Marti showed up.
> *Marti*—It's totally different from when I lived in Philly. We were constantly going to the local café ... going out more ... sorta being visible, sitting out on the stoop and talking or taking walks.
> *Marti*—I don't trust this neighborhood [Chester]. I feel ok now because people see me everyday, especially on this street. They see me, and people say hi and that's fine. I did feel very conspicuous ... you know, around here. I don't think it was an issue in West Philadelphia. There's basically people of ... everything, walking

around, doing their thing. And, I felt it was a more ... diverse place in general. So, I was very much an 'outside' person.

My other couple, Kevin in particular, seemed to feel his social personality affected their lack of public harassment. When asked is they had ever experienced physical violence, he answered in relation to his marriage. Kevin said:

> *Kevin*: No. We're very vanilla. Ya know, I can also add that that's part of my personality, though. I kinda blend in. I'm not one of those kinda people that's ...
> *Sarah*: In your face.
> *Kevin*: ahh ... yeah, out in the forefront there. So, probably that would account for why we've never had anything like that there.... that's a portion of it.

The researcher did observed differences in the neighborhoods of the two couples. Yngwie and Marti live in an area that is more than 80% Black. In contrast, Kevin and Sarah live in an area where there is much more diversity, including racial diversity. In commenting on their neighborhood, Kevin and Sarah said:

> *Kevin*: There's always a nice, ahh.... I'll say there's a broad spectrum of people ... variety.
> *Sarah*: Yeah, you kinda run the gamut from ...
> *Kevin*: Yeah ... there's some oddballs to ahh ...
> *Sarah*: There's some low-end and there's some high-end and we're all thrown in together ...
> *Kevin*: [to Sarah] Yeah, that's ever better. You got it.

There must be an aire of safety and security to their neighborhood. When using an avoidance strategy, the interracial couple may decide it is 'less trouble' for them to keep out of public places. Near the end of our discussion, Kevin did say, "In this area ... we rarely get to far away from here."

I discovered that Yngwie and Marti actually changed their travel plans due to an incident. They were a few days away from going to Colorado on vacation then, the Kobe Bryant incident occurred. They concluded it was in their interest, and personal safety, to vacation somewhere else:

> *Yngwie*—We went to Barbados instead of going to Colorado ... because the Kobe Bryant incident happened. We were going to Breckenridge and that's 10 minutes away and Marc Berger lives in Breckenridge, who's the DA. Also, there had just been an incident of neo-nazi's spreading propaganda about 'white women don't date Black men.' Any ya know, there have been no actual incidents, there been no ... but, its that thing of 'do I want to spend two-thousand dollars to drive across the country to feel uncomfortable?' Do I want to go on vacation and be looking over my shoulder?
>
> *Marti*—When you're going somewhere with the intention to relax, you don't want to be involved in a situation that could be ...
>
> *Yngwie*—She's gonna want to hiking and shit, and I'm gonna be like ... "What's That??" (What's that noise) ... oh ok, phew ... its just a mountain lion.
>
> *Yngwie*—I have no qualms about changing my travel plans to feel safe. I don't feel its necessary for me to take a stand, in that way. I'll take a stand and be like [sarcastically] 'we *gonna walk down the street in the middle of that KKK rally holdin hands, baby.*' Life's too short and I'm not interested. It's a big world and there are a lot of interesting places to go. I don't need to go someplace where I'm not going to feel safe.

Segregation

In segregation, people choose to enter or interact with people who are like them; with their own kind. Kevin and Sarah talked around finding people who are like them. For this couple, it could have more to do with geographic location (i.e. the over-crowdedness of Manhattan N.Y. vs. 'The Suburbs' of Philadelphia) than avoiding harassment:

Kevin: Because, when there is more space, you kinda ...
Sarah: Stand out more.
Kevin: Well, no. You tend to hang out with your 'like kind' ... people that are like you. You get to pick, that's it ... you can *pick* who you're gonna hang out with. You're forced to spend time with so many other people because there are so many people in such a small space.
Sarah: (while Kevin is talking, she says) You migrate to them because they are the only other Black person in the neighborhood.

Being Aware

In this research, the researcher came across other strategies that did not necessarily "fit" with the 6 strategies mentioned. In a separate study by Killian (2001), he also interviewed interracial couples about their lives together. In one section of his study, he mentioned how the white person of the couple did not look for, did not notice or were 'oblivious to' negative public reactions. The Black partner of the couple was found to be much more likely to notice harassment. For example, he asked a interracial couple 'who do you think is more sensitive to these kinds of looks and reactions?' The Black female responded, "Me. They look because, in a sense, I'm the problem. If he was with a white woman, no one would pay attention to him." (p.30).

In this study, the couples were asked if they noticed people reacting differently to them in public. After a moment of thought:

Sarah says to Kevin: I knew you were going to say you have, because I think you are hyper-aware of that.
Kevin: I pay a lot of attention to stuff but ...
Sarah: He's observant anyway.
Kevin: but ... the two of us ... see that kinda thing all the time.
Sarah: ... ya know, I can't say that I am really aware of that because I don't care. I guess if someone was really rude and obvious, I might obviously become aware of it but I don't kinda walk into somewhere and scan and see who's like ... doing a double take or ya know ... I really don't pay attention to that and I really don't let that alter my behavior any, so ...

In these comments, it is clear that Kevin is much more aware than Sarah. But at the same time, it is possible her level of awareness truly depends on the issue. For example during the interview, she was able to discern from a cacophony of various screams, that the crying child was not hers.

Fleeing

In doing this research, its is always important to remember that management strategies do not always work. In some cases, interracial couples are exposed to physical violence. Yngwie described a time when he was assaulted in Greece. He met a female (white) during his trip and decided to spend time with her in a area known as Praca. He continued:

> "... Praca is right below the Acropolis ... and there are all these shops and taverns and stuff. It's a bustling little area. And we're sitting below the Acropolis and there are all these ruins around, with digging going on. And umm ... these guys are sort of talking—I see them out of the corner of my eye and one of the walk to where the TV is (demonstrating that the guy is about 15 feet away from him); he comes in from the right, walks in front of me and then, walks back. And I had long hair at the time ... it was braids and he says *"einai arapis"* [Translation: "He's a nigger"], and I knew it wasn't anything ... he said it to his friends and they sort of chuckled. And, I knew it wasn't anything good but ... I just knew it was wrong some how. And the girl (her name is Evey)] said we should go. She starts packing up her lighter and cigarettes and my cigarettes, ya know, getting our stuff. So, we're walking and I realized she said "fascist." People in Europe always call skinhead "fascist," like it's a general term. So, we're walking as I was like 'well ok, we got away from them' cause we sort of ran into a crowd of people. Behind us, there were these ruins ... I guess where they were diggin. When they moved the rocks, they use these little cars and they have these little castors, and the castors have v-grooves in them so you can put them on a track. So, there are basically train tracks. So obviously, they had grabbed one of the (railroad) ties from the train track and they grabbed

some rocks. And the next thing I knew … I thought we had gotten rid of them … is I was smashed in the back of the head. And blood splattered out of my mouth … just all over … everywhere! It was sorta in slow motion, like "Bluahhhh" (demonstrating the blood ejecting from his mouth). And then, we just started running. We were holding hands and running and then, we got separated. And, there were chasin' after me and at the time, I was running a lot so, I out ran them. So, I ran and I ran. So, I stop and I look back and there was just one guy left and he was a little guy. So, it was just me and him and he had this one big rock so, we just stared at each other. So, he threw the rock … heaved the rock and I just sorta watched it go by. So, it was just me and him and he looked at me and he ran. So, I'm covered in blood and its everywhere so I had to walk back up the hill to find this girl, ya know … I cant just leave her. So, I start walking back up the hill and she's walking down the hill with a bunch of people who grabbed her … like, to hide her. They (the fascists) had actually kicked her and knocked her down and she rolled into a small area and they could not find her in the dark. They wanted to find her … cause they were screaming, ya know … 'Where's that bitch?' So then, we talked to the police who were absolutely no help at all. I remember screaming "HELP" and they were actually no help at all.

Conclusion

As you can see, the two couples I interviewed have had slightly different experiences with harassment. The one theme these couples commented on is geographic location. They both seem to feel they feel/felt safer in specific parts of the Delaware Valley. In the case of Yngwie and Marti, as a couple, they felt safer in West Philadelphia in contrast to his family's home in Chester. Kevin commented choosing that particular area to buy a home was affected by its location and the fact of his local social contacts.

Therefore, I tend to feel one of the more popular harassment strategy is avoiding—living away from possible harassment; choosing friends who are open-minded; changing travel plans to avoid possible harassment, etc.

What I also noticed the Black males are both aware. Even though I did not include a quote from Yngwie in that section, he did mention the possibility of being attacked in Colorado. I can say from my own experience, I was much more on guard when I was out in public. If I was surrounded by friends my guard would drop and I was able to have a good time. I can also add, when I was in an interracial relationship, I would never drink alcohol to the point of being drunk. I would "nurse" the same beer for hours while still remaining on guard. You never knew who was going to get drunk and change—they say the drunk tongue speaks the truth. So, there was always the possibility that someone who called himself or herself your friend would 'turn on you.'

I also realized, due to the small sample size of this research, my chance to gather a variety of stories was limited. For example, Marti mentioned to me if I had more time, I should have interviewed an interracial couple with whom she has contact. She mentioned they have experienced much more harassment. She told me that couple when to a meeting on Blacks and Education where a speaker told the audience 'we need to educate our Black men to stop marrying white women.' Yes, that other couple is comprised of a Black male and white female.

To end this research, I would like to see this same type of study completed on a much bigger sample. If someone would complete this same study with 40 couple, then the one could generalize the results to the public at large. I hope this was enlightening for the reader.

4

The Creation of The Homophobic Male

There are some people in this world who believe only their way is right. It is their way or the wrong way. This attitude is prevalent is many areas of life including international, interstate, and family relations. Since we live in patriarchical society, it is the male who is supposed to run the household. He is supposed to be dominant and heterosexual: the supreme achievement in a phallocentric society. Questions arise when a male enjoys the company and love of another male. Some of the heterosexual males resort to violence to state their feelings about a gay relationship. Who gives heterosexuals the right to force their sexual orientation onto another? This response may come from the 'majority rule' belief. Since gay males and lesbians are a minority in this country, heterosexuals believe they have the right to object violently to another persons way of life. Now, the question should be is heterosexuality or homosexuality natural?

In 1948, Alfred Kinsey released data which stated gay male and lesbian homosexuality accounted for ten percent of the adult population. He also found that the "incidence among single males rises in successive age groups until it reaches a maximum of 38.7 per cent between 36 and 40 years of age" (Kinsey et al., 1948, p.259). Does this mean there is a population of 'heterosexual' males who enjoy the company of another male? Is this a secret society of heterosexual males? These males must keep their affections for another male hidden due the patriarchical stereotype: a true man must have relations with a female. This should make you wonder what the life of a gay male or lesbian is like.

In this homophobic culture, being a homosexual is very trying. In 1982, only 45 percent of Americans felt homosexual relationships between consenting adults should be legal ("Public Perceptions of Gays", 1982). Added to this, 42.3 percent of college freshmen agreed with the statement "It is important to have laws prohibiting homosexual relationships" ("Freshman Survey", 1986). With such negative pressure reflecting public opinion, the mental stress must be unbearable. The research shows that heterosexual youth are two to three times less likely to attempt to end their life in contrast to homosexual children (Staff, 1990).

The AIDS epidemic has also affected the gay and lesbian life. Grossman (1991) believes there is a 'double stigma': Being gay, and at the same time, having the AIDS virus. Grossman is correct with his analysis. The research shows that gay males who have the AIDS virus are viewed as "less entitled for work, more deserving and responsible for his disease and, more deserving to die"p.95 (St. Lawrence et al, 1990). Where does this hated and fear come from? The purpose of this article is to show that the social scripts put forth by this culture help to create heterosexual males who will resort to violence when they feel their masculinity is threatened. This whole concept is maintained by patriarchy.

Development

Violence against gay men and lesbians in this country is increasing. The research shows more than ninety percent on gay men and seventy-five percent of lesbians have reported being verbally attacked just because of their sexuality. Additionally, almost fifty percent of gay males and one third of females have been threatened with physical violence just because of their sexual orientation. And worst of all, about twenty percent of gay men and almost ten percent of lesbians have reported they have been punched, hit, kicked, or beaten because of their homosexuality (National Gay Task Force, 1984). Reports from across the country state that such violence is increasing. It is gaining strength because of the AIDS epidemic and because of the perceived linkage between the epidemic and the 'gay lifestyle' (Greer, 1986; National Gay Task Force, 1988). One should ask where all of this hate and violence comes from. One important factor is how the males of this culture are socialized and how gender roles affect males.

Gender Roles

What is a gender role? Richmond-Abbott (1992 p.4) defined a gender role as a belief that "has come to mean entirely socially created expectations of masculine and feminine behavior." Like all of our other roles, gender roles are learned. Gender roles, like a tradition, are passed along from generation to generation.

In traditional gender roles, the man is the provider and the breadwinner. The female is supposed to be at home with the children and also, she has the job of keeping her husband happy. These traditional roles have been idealized for so long, they are just taken for granted as being normal. In traditional roles, the males are given a higher status. This also goes along with the patriarchal society in which we live. The next question should be who is teaching these roles an how are they learned?

According to the social learning theory, adults and children learn gender appropriate roles through interaction with the environment. An example would be a young female who is told she is cute for putting on make-up where a young male would be punished. Another example is when a young male is punished for crying and told 'big boys don't cry.' Males are socialized (taught) to be tough and unfeminine.

Gender roles are also learned through imitation or role modeling. Parents are seen as the major role models for children. Other role models can include care givers, friends and even television characters.

The social learning theory is useful for understanding the relationship between early learning processes and socializing methods. What causes young children to grow up and become violent and hateful toward gay males and lesbians?

Predictors

There are several reasons why these children grow up to become homophobic. Interestingly, the research shows heterosexual males hold the most anti-gay hatred on average than do heterosexual women (Kite, 1984). This issue will be addressed later in the article.

Herek (1984a) did research in the area of homophobia focusing on the social and psychological correlates. He found, in contrast to people with liberal attitudes, heterosexual with conservative attitudes are: 1) more likely to show traditional attitudes about gender roles; 2) more likely to hold higher levels of authoritarianism and related behaviors; 3) more likely to see their peers as having negative attitudes towards homosexuals; 4) less likely to have had personal contact with a gay man or lesbian; and 5) more likely to believe and follow a conservative religious ideology.

Other research has found that people who live in the south are more conservative on homosexual issues (Hulbert, 1989). Additionally, a national study was done on 15 to 19 year old males to state their attitudes toward homosexuals. The research showed that eighty-nine percent of the males felt sexual behavior between two men was "disgusting". Also, fifty-nine percent said they could not even be friends with a gay person (Marsiglio, 1993). The same study also found the subjects were less likely to have a gay friend when their parent(s) had finished fewer years of school. The researcher believes the young males are learning their intolerance based on their parent(s) educational (the way the parents own values and beliefs were formed) experiences (Marsiglio, 1993). What causes males to progress from ignorance to violence?

Homophobic Social Roles

In this culture, males have defined social roles. Since male sex role behaviors are more visible (defined) thus, more threatening, males are judged more harshly for 'abnormal' behavior (Rushing, 1979). The data shows gender nonconformity is judged more seriously in males than in females (Page, Yee, 1986). To add, Herek (1986) believes since this country emphasizes the importance of heterosexuality with masculinity, many males feel the need to reaffirm their masculinity by rejecting males who 'violate' the heterosexual norm. This 'anxiety' comes from their fear of losing their sense of self as a true heterosexual man. Herek (1986) concluded that:

> "Conformity to social standards and defense against anxiety push heterosexual men to express homophobic attitudes and provide rewards in the form of social support and reduced anxiety, both of which increase self-esteem. In other words, heterosexual men reaffirm their male identity by attacking gay men" (p. 567).

Since heterosexuality needs to be 'protected', why aren't heterosexual women attacking lesbians? The research shows that some people view female homosexuality as being closer to normality, or less abnormal, than male homosexuality (Page, Yee, 1986). This could be related to gender roles. Since heterosexual females are less likely to see homosexuals as an important part of their gender identity, in contrast to heterosexual males, they probably experience fewer social influences to cause the development of a hostile attitude.

Conclusion

The point of this article was to provide insight that social roles and how they are passed along help to contribute to the creation of a homophobic male and a homophobic society. This culture has several events that must be changed before everyone is seen as equal. First, it is necessary for people to be allowed to discover their sexuality without the influence of a esoteric variable. This variable is called patriarchy. Maintaining a heterosexual culture helps to buttress male patriarchy. This culture says there are bonuses for getting in line and following society. One of the bonuses for being a heterosexual is dominating a female: 'If you follow us, you get to control a family and pass your beliefs (family values) onto your children.'

Secondly, with the fall of patriarchy, no one will be threatened by another's' sexual orientation. Therefore, the amount of violence toward gays and lesbians would sharply decrease. I am sure patriarchy will still be around in my lifetime but I can do what I can to get rid of it. I can vote in people who are in line with the idea of creating a society of equals and the elimination of discrimination.

It is important to also look at what is likely to happen if nothing is done to change this homophobic society. The violence against homosexuals is likely to increase. I predict the people who hold up signs saying 'Kill a Fag' will probably put down the sign and pick up a bat or gun. With people like Senator Phil Gramm, the anti-gay poster boy, spouting his rhetoric against homosexuals and the 'gay lifestyle,' it is only a matter of time before the violence escalates. Do not forget, the homophobic people are looking for a leader and he may be the one. An interesting study would be to look for a correlation between senator Gramm's anti-gay speeches and the increase in violence against homosexuals. But, there are other sources of attacks against homosexuals.

How does religious teaching play into the homophobic society. Pat Robertson is the leader of the Christian Coalition, a Christian political group and think-tank. They believe there is a 'gay agenda' that involves the moral corruption of the fabric of America. This 'gay agenda' also involves the conversion of heterosexuals to homosexuals and turning their children into sexual perverts. The 700 Club, a popular program from their television network, constantly shows gay parades. The camera is always focused on the most extreme and outrageous people of the bunch ... men wearing dresses and gay and lesbian couples kissing, checking each other for loose bridgework. It would seem to be the religious right is more obsessed with the 'gay lifestyle' than actual homosexuals. Question: what exactly is the gay lifestyle? If you asked a gay person and a member of the Christian Coalition, I am positive you would get two completely different answers.

In this homophobic society, who would a homosexual be more likely to come out to? A person who was highly educated, politically liberal and female (Herek, Glunt, 1993). Why? Because this person is less likely to respond in a negative manner. This is called selective disclosure: homosexuals voluntarily disclose their sexual orientation to a heterosexual from whom they would expect a positive response (Wells, Kline, 1987).

I have a possible topic for research. Since, I stated earlier, heterosexual females are less likely than heterosexual males to be threatened by lesbians, who is harassing lesbians? Males. It would have to be. My thesis would be that heterosexual males see lesbians as an object they can never dominate. Therefore, males harass lesbians because it is in direct conflict with their socialization (gender role). Heterosexual males probably say things like 'if you spend the night with me, I could change you over'. In this instance, there seems to be a 'straight (heterosexual) agenda'. It is called Patriarchy.

5

Issues Affecting the Lives of Gays and Lesbians

Is America the land of equal opportunity? That depends on who you talk to. Some people are fired because they are just not productive people. Interestingly enough, a population of people are fired because of their sexual orientation. 'We don't want any gays around here' or 'You people are sick and you should have no right to work in this occupation'. These statements are probably heard more by people who are gay and lesbian. What causes this form of discrimination?

There are populations of people in this country who believe they are better than other sbased on things ranging from the color of a person's skin to whom they choose to fall in love with. Who says only one way of life is correct? This belief is based on and supported by patriarchy: the belief that males (heterosexual, white) make the rules for this society.

Therefore, anyone stepping outside on these boundaries are defined as being deviant. The issue of 'majority rule' is used to support the actions of people who support patriarchy. This rule gives these people the right to discriminate and become violent toward someone *they* define as deviant.

When gays and lesbians are forced to survive under these conditions, how can someone expect to live a full and rewarding life? Staying in the closet is an option but, being secretive about everything must be harming socially. But, one cannot maintain any form of a 'healthy' life with no employment or income. While some people in this country are allowed to express themselves openly, others are forced to live in silence.

This paper focuses on two areas that affect the lives of gays and lesbians: Violence and Discrimination. It should be noted parts of this paper were focused on lesbians because the author felt his knowledge of this area was lacking. Violence and discrimination are two major issues that effect the lives of gays and lesbians but, by no means are these the only two issues.

This paper is based on explorational literature searches. The author wishes this article to enlighten the readers to try to understand how violence and discrimination impacts the lives of gay and lesbian people. Hopefully, the readers will begin to question their own attitudes and behaviors toward gays and lesbians. If you are not part of the solution then, you are part of the problem!

Development

Violence

Violence against gays and lesbians is increasing. Depending on the study, some research shows that more than half of the respondents have reported violence due to their sexual orientation (Comstock, 1989). This same report states that more men report victimization than women and a higher level of violence is reported by gays and lesbians of color (Comstock, 1989).

Students in places of higher education are not safe. It has been reported between fifty-five and seventy-two percent of gays and lesbians have been the recipient of some form of physical or verbal abuse (D'Augelli, 1992). In this same study, it was found that the highest rate, sixty-four percent, of abuse came from the subject's roommate. Surprisingly, it was also noted that twenty-three percent of abusers were the school faculty, staff and administrators (D'Augelli, 1992).

In a report compiled by the Anti-Violence Project (AVP) of New York City, they found violence towards gays and lesbians increased eight percent in the city of New York and two percent nationwide. The report looked at 151 murders in twenty-nine states. They found almost sixty percent of the murders involved "forensic overkill," where the victim was "butchered." In twenty-four cases, the victim was stabbed more than twelve times. In twenty-four percent of attacks, multiple weapons were used. Their data also found that when the victims are "overkilled," racism still plays a part. Seventy-one percent of Latino/a victims and sixty-three percent of African-American victims experienced "overkill" compared to fifty-two percent of white victims (New York Gay and Lesbian Anti-Violence Project, 1995). With all the violence on the streets, gays and lesbians are still subject to violence within their own personal relationships.

There has been research looking at violence in lesbian relationships. Out of 284 lesbians surveyed, ninety percent have been involved in one or more acts of verbal aggression from their partners. (Lockhard et al., 1994). This research found that the majority of the aggressive acts were caused by conflicts involving money, emotional dependency, housekeeping and sexual activities. Thirty-one percent of the subjects reported physical abuse with the relationship. Physical abuse was likely to be triggered by 1) questions of power in the relationship and 2) the level of independent and interdependence with in the relationship (Lockhard et al., 1994). It would be interesting to note how alcohol affects gay and lesbian relationships.

It has been found that between twenty and thirty-three percent of the people who consider themselves to be gay or lesbian have a drinking problem (Kus, 1990). To support this data, research found that approximately one-third of lesbians abuse alcohol (Fifeld, 1980). This percentage is higher than the general population whose drinking problem was estimated between ten and twelve percent (Gosselin, Nice, 1987). One should ask if there is a relationship between the use of alcohol and violence in lesbian relationships?

In the heterosexual population, Frieze and Knoble (1980) reported a correlation of .24 between drinking in battered women and drinking and their spouses. This finding suggests the incidence of alcohol abuse may be higher in violent situations where the partner also drinks (Frieze, Knoble, 1980). To support this data, it was found that the victim's use of alcohol was significant to the differences between batterers and non-batterers (Eberle, 1982). To bring this idea full circle, there is research that reveals sixty-four percent of both batterers and victims, in lesbian relationships, report using alcohol and other drugs prior to or during the incidents of battering (Schilit et al., 1990). One should ask why is the frequency of alcohol abuse so high in the lesbian population?

Isolation and oppression are parts of life that lesbians have to deal with. Therefore, it is believed that may lesbians are finding an 'escape' with alcohol and other drugs (Anderson, Henderson, 1985). It has been observed that alcohol use among lesbians is related to 1) feelings of low self esteem, 2) depression, 3) anger, 4) frustration, 5) isolation, 6) problems of a sexual nature and 7) the social environment of lesbian bars (Burke, 1982).

It is also believed the use of alcohol may aid the person in the "coming out" process (Nardi, 1982). During this process, an unusual amount of stress may be created and the alcohol is used to relieve the stress. Also, the use of alcohol may lower the person's inhibitions as a way to aid them to perform in same-sex sexual activities (Israelstam. Lambert, 1984).

Discrimination

To add insult to injury, gays and lesbians have to put up with the constant obstacle of discrimination. It seems that the culture supports the discrimination of gays and lesbians through the use of stereotypes. It was found that sixty-two percent of Americans feel the homosexual orientation is a curable illness; seventy-four percent feel homosexuals are dangerous as teachers because they will try to get sexually involved with children; thirty-nine percent feel homosexuals would corrupt fellow workers; fifty-nine percent feel homosexuals have unusually strong sex drives; and sixty-nine percent feel homosexuals act like the other sex (Levitt, Klassen, 1974).

To add, research found that the majority of people supported barring gays from 'high status' jobs. Seventy-seven percent of the study felt gays should not be allowed to be court judges, school teachers or ministers. Sixty-eight percent opposed allowing gays work as medical doctors and government officials (Levitt, Klassen, 1974).

A Gallup poll (1977) found information that lends support for this research. Sixty-five percent of the public was opposed to gays teaching in elementary schools; fifty-four percent was opposed to gays working as clergy; forty-four percent opposed gay doctors; and thirty-three percent opposed gay military personnel.

In contrast, the research found that these people had little opposition to gays working in 'lower status' jobs. Twenty-eight percent were against employment as a beautician. Sixteen percent were against gay workers as artists, fifteen percent were against gay workers as musicians and only thirteen percent were against gays working as florists (Levitt, Klassen, 1974). Since there are parts of the population who believe gays and lesbians should not work in certain, well paying areas, how does a gay or lesbian retain the capacity to be discriminated against?

It was hypothesized by Goffman (1963) that there are two kinds of sexual stigmas which help to maintain this discrimination. The first stigma has to do with the ability to *discredit* the person: the gay or lesbian who is publicly known by their own admission or by official record. The second stigma has to do with the person who is *discreditable*: those gays and lesbians who "pass" and keep their sexual orientation a secret from the non-gay world. Even, the hiring agencies themselves get in the way of employment.

It was observed that some of the employment agencies have set up special codes for the employers. On the resumes of "suspected homosexuals," the agency writes the code "H.C.F"= High Class Fairy (Zoglin, 1974). With this kind of discrimination, the effects on the lives of gay and lesbian people far exceed just the area of employment.

Due to the impact of discrimination, gay and lesbians have been forced to change their career goals. Many are forced into jobs and situations they are overqualified or just do not want to be a part of:

> "My goals are affected. I have to choose a job where I won't be discriminated against (Bell, Weinberg, 1978).
> "Homosexuality forced me out of the service and caused me to become a hairdresser because here only I could be myself (Saghir, Rabins, 1974).

Lesbian Discrimination

Just as gay males are subject to employment discrimination, lesbians are subject to the same hostile environment. Chafetz (1974) found most lesbians feared losing their jobs. Sixty percent felt the possibility of losing their jobs if their sexual orientation was made public. These fears have relevance because the research reveals that twelve percent were asked to resign, or were fired or were given warnings when their sexual orientation was made public (Saghir, Robins, 1973). In what ways do lesbians deal with their work situation?

Bell and Weinberg (1978) found that most lesbians hid their sexual orientation while on the job, with sixty percent hiding it from employers and almost half hiding their sexual orientation from fellow workers. More resent research shows that seventy-seven percent were partially or totally closeted on the job: twenty-nine percent told some friends, twenty-one percent told only people they considered close friends and twenty-seven percent told no one at all (Levine, Leonard, 1984). Since there is a population of people who do not want gays and lesbians in high status jobs (or close to children), how do some principals feel about gay and lesbian teachers?

As I stated earlier, Levitt and Klassen (1974) found that forty-five percent of their sample felt that gay and lesbian teachers for young children were dangerous. They also found that seventy-five percent of their sample would deny gays and lesbians the right to choose teaching as a career. In 1985, Dressler reported findings from a questionnaire. This questionnaire was sent to the principals of high schools around the country. The main findings of this research were: 1) the principals supported the action of loss of license in 'non-sexual conduct circumstances' if the teacher was active in political "gay rights" activities, and 2) the majority of the principals concluded that a teacher was gay or lesbian based on rumor, stereotypical thinking, or guilt by association (Dressler, 1985). To build on this theme, since part of the population does not approve of the idea and principles hold reservations toward gay and lesbian teachers, how do gay and lesbian teachers survive when they choose this career?

Interviews were conducted by Olson (1987) with gay and lesbian teachers. These teachers were posed several questions. *What kept you from being open?* The majority of responses were that the teachers wanted acceptance from superiors and peers, and these teachers feared loosing their jobs or not receiving tenure or promotions.

What do you feel that you had to offer education that was unique because of your sexual preference? Almost half felt they were more "sensitive to differences" because of their minority sexual orientation. Several others said they had become more "feeling" and they could relate to the needs of their students.

In what ways do (did) you find to survive the prejudicial treatment leveled against you as a gay teacher? Finding other gay and lesbian teachers for support was the most frequent response given. Others said they preferred to stay "in the closet" (see above citations).

What do you feel can be done to make educators more sensitive to gay or lesbian issues? About thirty-three percent felt that more homosexual teachers need to come out of the closet as a way to build more trust (Olson, 1987). It should be interesting to note that discrimination against teachers is not confined to this country only. In Canada, a law was passed in order to help gay and lesbian teachers get some form of equality in their profession.

On December 2, 1986, the Legislature of Ontario passed Bill 7, Section 15 of the Ontario Human Rights Code which made it illegal to deny anyone employment, housing or services on the basis of sexual orientation. This was viewed as a very positive step forward for equal rights for gays and lesbians of Canada but, it did not cure all the problems gays and lesbians face.

There are unwritten rules that society lives by. "A lesbian teacher cannot be tolerated, not just because her existence would negate the myth that female sexuality does not exists irrespective of men ... (but), her sexuality must be reflective of the official ideology" (Khayatt, 1990). Could this be the social construction of heterosexuality?

It is believed by this author that the people in the Ontario Legislature felt the passage of Bill 7 would be a 'cure all' for the social problems gays and lesbians went through. Some interviews with lesbian teachers reveal their true thoughts about this issue:

> "... even though there is legislation on paper, which is an important first step, there still is not the social acceptance". p.189
> "I would have to dig back into the recesses of my mind to remember what Bill 7 is. That's how much of a difference it has made in my life". (Khayatt, 1990, p.189)

Conclusion

The purpose of this paper was to shed light on specific issues that affect the lives of gays and lesbian. Think about it. When you are gay or a lesbian, you have to live in fear and constantly look over your shoulder. What kind of life is this? People say living in America is great because of all the "freedoms" we have but, to be realistic, gays and lesbians are confined to their own individual prison.

There are some people who are against equal rights for gays and lesbians. Even if a law was passed that said it was illegal to discriminate against gays and lesbians, unless there is a reconstruction of the culture, the discrimination will continue. We can use Bill 7 of Canada as an example. The mental strain of trying to survive in a homophobic culture must be overwhelming.

To be gay or lesbian in this culture means you cannot be yourself. In other words, you cannot live, you have to learn to survive. With the constant threat of being fired from your job, beaten up or 'over-killed', you have to develop an 'aire' of distrust because you have no way of knowing how certain people will react to your sexual orientation. And also, if you find someone who you can love, there is no guarantee that relationship will not become violent and threaten your general health. So, as a culture, how can we end the violence gays and lesbians experience out in the 'streets' as well as the violence in the home?

Well, I am a social constructionist. I believe education is the key. It is necessary for teachers who are gay or lesbian to come out. This way, the children will know they are capable of loving someone just like everyone else. They just love people who are of their same sex. This could also be a way of gaining respect. When John Anderson (1994) was talking to a friend, he said "… we gay and lesbians would have to gain acceptance on an individual basis."

I know the religious right will not agree with me at all. But, it seems to me they are a bunch of hypocrites. They say 'God created everyone equal' but, since gays and lesbians cannot procreate, there must be an unwritten rule which says '… unless you love someone of the same sex'! I wonder if the religious right would dare say God made a mistake?

Then, there also must be changes in how treat victims of violence. When a person goes in to seek therapy, the counselor must be sensitive to the needs of the victim. If the counselor is uneducated with the daily lives of gays and lesbians, more harm than good could come out of the counseling secession. To begin, if the gay or lesbian victim does not feel this is a 'safe place', the therapy will end even before it begins.

How could we end employment discrimination against gays and lesbians? It would seem to me if you got rid of the discrimination first, the end of the violence would soon follow. It seems that both discrimination and violence are both supported by homophobia. Homophobia gets the majority of its strength for patriarchy. Now, it would be a great day when the gay and lesbian organizations as well as the women of this country, at the same time, demanded equal rights. If you want to change this culture, this is how to do it. Since this is not likely to happen, it is necessary to keep an eye on certain politicians and this current presidential race. It is important to ask yourself what would happen if there was a republican congress as well as a new republican president?

Just recently, a few of the contestants for the republican nomination to run against Clinton signed a statement which says they will outlaw same-sex marriages. If these people get into office, I am positive they will not stop there. The Christian Coalition would probably try to lobby ideas that have an even greater effect on the lives of gays and lesbians in this country. It is possible that a bill would be brought up before congress which states something like 'it is illegal for gays and lesbians to teach in Americas' schools.' This is why it is necessary for the people of this country to look at these presidential candidates with a magnifying class to expose their real hidden agendas.

6

Research Issues Regarding Sexual Orientation

Should researchers measure sexual orientation on a continuum or should bisexuals, gays and lesbians be studied as specific groups? Do researchers view sexual orientation as a choice or are individuals born as gays or lesbians? Kinsey et al. (1948) used a continuum scale and found 37% of the men had at least one same-gender sexual experience; 13% had same-gender sexual fantasies but no actual sexual behavior while, 10% had primarily same-gender sexual experiences during adolescence. So, what does this research really mean? Without an accepted theoretical construct or specific definition, research on sexual orientation leaves much open to speculation.

Definition

Today, the terminology heterosexual (straight), homosexual (gay and lesbian), and bisexual are the more universal used terms used by scientists and educators to describe sexual orientations (Sell and Petrulio, 1995). There have been new terms created to describe heterosexuality and bisexuality. Many terms have been used by researchers to describe homosexuality, including uranianism, homogenic love, contrasexuality, homo-erotism, similsexualism, tribanism sexual inversion, intersexuality, transexuality, third sex and psychosexual hermaphroditism

(Ulrichs, 1994; Moll, 1891; Carpenter, 1894; Ellis and Symonds, 1896; Mayne, 1908; Kinsey et al., 1948, 1953). Looking at today's more common term of 'sexual orientation,' it has a variety of definitions while these are usually made of one or two components: a "psychological" component and a "behavioral" component.

Looking historically, Mayne's (1908) definition of the term *Urning* and Benkert's use of the term *homosexual* (Robinson, 1936) mainly focused on the description of the psychological state. Mayne's definition focused on how an individuals feelings regarding sexual passion determined their sexual orientation while Benkert mentioned a sort of sexual "urge." Ellis also mentioned a psychological entity that he described as a "sexual instinct." Ellis defined homosexuality as a "sexual instinct turned by inborn constitution abnormality toward persons of the same sex" (Ellis and Symonds, 1896). Many of these early definitions exclude any discussions of behavior. Krafft-Ebing (1886), just like his peers, decided to keep sexual behavior out of the definition of homosexuality. Krafft-Ebing felt that "the determining factor here is the demonstration of perverse feelings for the same sex; not the proof of sexual acts with the same sex. These two phenomena must not be confounded with each other."

When looking at some of the more current factors of the psychological definition, it is important to note the variations within. Some definitions of the psychological component may include terms like "sexual passion," "sexual urge," "sexual feelings," "sexual attraction," "sexual interest," "sexual arousal," "sexual desire," "affectional preference," "sexual instinct," "sexual orientation identity," and "sexual preference." Each of these phrases has a specific meaning but may not represent the exact same experience (Sell, 1997).

Golden (1987) created a multi-dimensional model for defining a homosexual orientation. First, the individual must identify him/herself as a homosexual. Secondly, the individual must have sexual behaviors that include same-sex activities. Third, the individual must participate in the gay/lesbian community. So, what would a person "be" if they (1) did not identify as gay/lesbian, (2) engaged in same-sex sexual behaviors and (3) was a wavering member of the gay/lesbian community?

The APA Committee on Lesbian and Gay Concerns (CLGC) came up with recommendations for language concerning gays and lesbians. To aid in understanding, the CLGC (1991) presented this statement:

> "The terms gay male and lesbian refer primarily to identities and to the modern culture and communities that have developed among people who share those identities. They should be distinguishing from sexual behavior. Some men and women have sex with others of their own gender but do not consider themselves to be gay or lesbian."

Other researchers felt that sexual behavior plays a major part in the definition of homosexuality. For example, Beach (1950) said that "the term {homosexuality} means different things to different people ... it is preferable to set forth the significance of the term as used in this discussion. Homosexuality refers exclusively to overt behavior between two individuals of the same sex. The behavior must be patently sexual, involving erotic arousal and, in most instances at least, resulting in the satisfaction of the sexual urge" (cited in Sell, 1997, p, 648). To add, Diamond (1993) felt this type of behavioral definition is supported by scientists and researchers to aid in determining the size of the "homosexual" population in diverse countries. In the studies reviewed by Diamond, he noted all of the research on homosexuality used some measure of sexual behavior to measure the prevalence of sexual orientation but none of them used any measure of an individual's psychological sexual attraction.

Once again, there are variations within the various terms used to define the behavioral component. When looking at behavior, it can be called something as general as "sexual behavior," or can it be called "genital activity," "sexual contact," or "sexual contact that achieves orgasm?" Sell (1997) asks the question to researchers regarding how one would actually define these terms for scientific measurement.

One of the more recent definitions of homosexuality includes both components, behavioral and psychological. LeVay (1993) defined sexual orientation as "the direction of sexual feelings or behavior toward individuals of the opposite sex (heterosexuality), the same sex (homosexuality), or some combination of the two (bisexuality). Further, Weinrich (1994) defined homosexuality "either (1) as a genital act or (2) as a long-term sexuerotic status." In these definitions, the psychological conditions are called 'sexual feelings' and 'sexuoerotic status,' while the behavioral result is LeVey's 'sexual feelings' and Weinrich's 'genital act.' The use of the conjunction "*or*" shows that either component can be used to measure a person's sexual orientation (Sell, 1997).

Operational Measures

The measurement of an individual's sexual orientation is important to the research on gay, lesbian and bisexuals. Without an accurate understanding of people's orientation, the researchers do not have accurate knowledge regarding their sample. A study by Shively, Jones and DeCecco (1984) reviewed 228 articles on gays, lesbians and bisexuals. Their results found in 81% of the articles reviewed, an individual's sexual orientation was assumed rather than actually measured, which raises questions about the validity of the early research. More importantly, there is no agreement about how sexual orientation should be measured (Berkey, Perelman-Hall & Kurdek, 1990). It seems that various theories recommend different assessment methods but the topic of actually operationally defining sexual orientation has been ignored (Klein, Sepekoff & Wolf, 1985).

Looking historically, some of the earliest information on measuring sexual orientation came from documents of the Western Church, where people were encouraged to admit their sins. These documents revealed the church was interested in questioning people about topics that included same-sex behaviors (Lee, 1993; Tentler, 1977).

De Pareja went to Florida as a missionary for the Timucua Indians in 1595. While there, he had certain questions to detect sodomites in his book, *Confessionario* (Katz, 1992). Some of the questions in the book included:

1. Have you had intercourse with another man?

2. Have you gone around trying out or making fun in order to do that?

3. Has someone been investigating you from behind?

4. Did you consummate the act? (Katz, 1992).

In 1908, Mayne, created a series of hundreds of questions for the diagnosis of "Urings" and "Urningins." Some of the questions included:

1. At what age did you sexual desire show itself distinctly?

2. Did it direct itself at first most to the male or to the female sex? Or, did it hesitate awhile between both?

3. Is the instinct unvaryingly toward the male or female sex now?—or do you take pleasure (or would you experience it) with now a man, now a woman?

4. Do you give away to it rather mentally or physically? Or are both in equal measure?

5. Is the semilsexual desire constant, periodic or irregularly felt?

6. In dreams, do you have visions of sexual relations with men or women, the more frequently and ardently?

Therefore, in looking at the possible choices of answers for these questions, the respondents were expected to give yes or no answers. In other words, the respondents were going to be categorized as a "Sodomite," "Urning," "Urningin" or not. So it seems that this basic method of classification of sexual orientation is still used by researchers today. The subjects of research are classified as homosexual or heterosexual based on their sexual identity or sexual behavior (Sell & Petrulio, 1995).

Chung and Katayama (1996) reviewed methods for assessing sexual orientation in 144 articles published in the Journal of Homosexuality. Their research found 33% of the publications used "self-identification" as an assessment method. Shively and Dececco (1977) a person's sexual identity is created from four factors: biological sex, gender identity, social sex-role, and sexual orientation. These authors suggest using "self-identification" as a measurement tool may be more telling about a persons sexual identify versus their orientation. Secondly, while a persons sexual orientation is said to be stable (Silverstein, 1997), a persons sexual identity can vary depending on their identity development (Cass, 1983).

From the Chung and Katayama study, they found that a "single dimension" method was used in 12.5% of the publications. The first problem with this method was that it fails to account for the variable aspects of sexual orientation (i.e. Kinsey Scale) (Coleman, 1987; Klein et al., 1985). Secondly, another critique is that heterosexuality and homosexuality are treated as two ends on a continuum. Storms (1978) suggested that homosexuality and heterosexuality may be separate, independent dimensions versus a uni-dimensional factor.

Finally, the Chung and Katayama (1996) study found that sexual behavior was an assessment factor used in 9% of the publications. They suggest, due to social oppression, a homosexual may engage in a heterosexual relationship or, if the person in truly bisexual, they may engage in a heterosexual/homosexual relationship which does not embody their 'real' orientation. Secondly, Blumstein and Schwartz (1976) did not find a correlation between a person's sexual behavior and their self-identification. Also, Bell and Weinberg (1978) found low correlations between a person sexual behavior and their erotic fantasies.

Aside from classifying individuals by their identity or behavior, one of the other more common methods for assessing orientation includes sexual fantasies (Sell & Petrulio, 1995) which can also be problematic. Klein et al., (1985) created the Kline Sexual Orientation Grid (KDOG). This tool measures seven factors including sexual attraction, sexual behavior, sexual fantasies, emotional preference, social preference, self-identification and heterosexual/homosexual lifestyle. One of the major issues with this scale appears when measuring many factors that are added to an overall score. This scale becomes heavier/denser and less useful for many research applications. This is one reason why many researchers tend to reduce the number of measured factors (Sell, 1997).

One of the more significant scales develop to measure sexual orientation was created by Kinsey et al., (1948, 1953) in their publication on sexual behavior in the human male and female. Kinsey and company produced a bipolar scale that allowed for a range between "exclusive heterosexuality" and "exclusive homosexuality." The Kinsey group wrote the following rationalization regarding their decision to reject the *either/or* models of their predecessors:

> "The world is not to be divided into sheep and goats. Not all things are black nor all things white. It is a fundamental of taxonomy that nature rarely deals with discrete categories. Only the human mind invents categories and tries to force facts into separated pigeon-holes. The living world is a continuum in each and every one of its aspects. The sooner we learn this concerning human sexual behavior the sooner we shall reach a sound understanding of the realities of sex" (Kinsey et al., 1948).
>
> "It is characteristic of the human mind that it tries to dichotomize in its classification of phenomena. Things are either so, or they are not so. Sexual behavior is either normal or abnormal, socially acceptable or unacceptable, heterosexual or homosexual; and many persons do not want to believe that there are gradations

in these matters from one to the other extreme" (Kinsey et al., 1953).

One of the major critiques is that the Kinsey Scale forces individuals into one of seven categories. Secondly, it is difficult to measure people into a specific number when there are an infinite number of points on the continuum. For example, an individual has the chance to end up with a score of 2.3885 on the Kinsey scale. So, what does that really mean? Further, Masters and Johnson (1979) provided the following critiques in using the Kinsey scale:

> "There was also concern in arbitrarily selecting the specific classification of Kinsey grades 2 though 4 for any individual who has had a large number of both homosexual and heterosexual experiences. The ratings were assigned by the research team after detailed history-taking, but it is difficult for any individual to be fully objective in assessing the amounts of his or her heterosexuality versus homosexual experience when there has been a considerable amount of both types of interaction. Some of these preferences ratings might well be subject to different interpretations by other health-care professionals."

Another issue with the Kinsey scale is that it improperly measures homosexuality and heterosexuality on the same scale, making one "trade-off" the other. For example, later research on masculinity and femininity noted that the notions of masculinity and femininity are more correctly measured as unrelated concepts on different scales in contrast to being lumped together and measured on a single continuum with each concept representing opposite extremes (Bem, 1981). With both concepts measured on the same scale, an individual has to be more feminine in order to be less masculine *or* to be more masculine, one has to be less feminine. Being measured on separate scales, an individual could be both very masculine and very feminine (androgynous) or not very much other either (undifferentiated) (Sell, 1997). To add, when looking at homosexuality and heterosexuality on separate scales opens the possibility for an individual to be very heterosexual and very homosexual (bisexual) or not very much of either (Bullough, 1990).

Two of the early supporters for measuring homosexuality and heterosexuality on separate scales were Shively and DeCecco. They felt when homosexuality and heterosexuality were calculated separately, the degree of homosexuality and heterosexuality can be independently measured. Shively and DeCecco (1977) created a five-point scale where heterosexuality and homosexuality were measured separately. In using their scale, they suggested the measurement of two factors of sexual orientation: physical and affectional preference.

Storms (1980) measured the amounts of homosexual fantasies and heterosexual fantasies on two separate scales. He found that bisexuals were just as likely to report homosexual fantasies as homosexuals to report homosexual fantasies, and bisexuals were just as likely to report heterosexual fantasies as heterosexual were to report heterosexual fantasies. From this research he concluded, using the idea that bisexuals should be less likely to report homosexual fantasies than homosexuals, and less likely to report heterosexual fantasies than heterosexuals, that homosexuality and heterosexuality should be measured separately.

Development of Orientation

With so many sexual behaviors, attitudes and identities, researchers are questioning their origins. Research by Money (1987) suggested the importance of social and biological factors. In the 1990's, attention broadened to other possible causes of sexual orientation (LeVey, 1993). More specifically, much attention moved toward the possible genetic causes of sexual orientation (Bailey et al., 1995). But still, others are interested in development of sexual orientation and its timing of appearance.

In looking at childhood and family relationships, Thompson et al. (1973) recorded several differences between heterosexual and homosexual. The behaviors that were most likely to distinguish heterosexual woman from lesbians included (a) playing baseball, (b) being more athletic, (c) did not play with girls before adolescence, and (d) engaged in more physical fights. Gay men were (a) less likely to have played baseball or (b) other competitive games, (c) felt less accepted by father, (d) were more frail and clumsy, (e) did not play with boys before adolescence and (f) were more likely to be the center of mother's attention. Gays also reported being anxious about physical injury and also avoided physical fights. Thompson et al. (1973) also felt that "Alienation ... and a psychology of differences characterize both male and female homosexuals in this sample" (p.126).

In 1979, Troiden develop a sequence for gay males to accept their orientation as a part of their identity. The first stage is called *sensitization*, which begins before puberty and is distinguished by general perceptions of being different from same-sex peers. The second stage, *identity confusion*, appears when the individual experiences confusion which is related to negative social stigma, same-sex behavior and being socially isolated. The third stage, *identity assumption*, is when the individual beings to examine their life experiences through a lens of a homosexual. The final stage in the Troiden (1979) model, *commitment*, refers to the individual's self-acceptance and security with the homosexual identity and role.

Also in 1979, Cass created a stage model of homosexual identity formation. In this model, the concept is that an individual's sexual identity appears when they encounter incongruity between their perceptions about a characteristic they attributed to themselves; their perceptions of the behavior; and the beliefs on how others perceive them. The individual's attempts to create congruity with these factors lead them through a chain of separate steps. These steps are Identity Confusion, Identity Comparison, Identity Tolerance, Identity Acceptance, Identity Pride and Identity Synthesis. Cass (1979) also felt, at any stage, the individual could choose to stop, where Identity Foreclosure happens. To explain the stages in more detail:

- Identity Confusion—in this stage, the individual develops an awareness that homosexuality is relevant to themselves and their behavior; notices inconsistencies between self-perception of heterosexuality and the perceptions of others' that the individual is heterosexual.

- Identity Comparison—the individual notices social alienation while other perceives them to be heterosexual while questioning their own homosexuality and sexual behaviors.

- Identity Tolerance—this stage is related to the increasing commitment to a homosexual self-perception and a tendency to seek out the homosexual subculture.

- Identity Acceptance—the individual increases contact with homosexuals, allowing themselves to judge homosexuality more positively; passing as a heterosexual becomes more difficult.

- Identity Pride—this step involves the individuals issue in dealing the positive perceptions of the self as homosexual and society's negative perception of homosexuality; tend to reject heterosexual society.

- Identity Synthesis—this is the final stage where the individual encounters positive interactions with heterosexuals and understands that the idea of 'good' homosexuals and 'bad' heterosexuals is inaccurate.

A study by Halpin and Allen (2004) used the Cass model to study gay men through their relationship orientation development and psychosocial variables, which included happiness-sadness, satisfaction with life, self-esteem, and loneliness. They found these relationships were not linear as predicted. Actually, they were more of a "U" shape meaning greater levels of distress were associated with the middle stages—Identity tolerance and Identity acceptance. The early stages of Identity pride and Identity comparison were similar to the later stages of Identity pride and Identity synthesis showing fairly low levels of distress.

Halpin and Allen (2004) concluded that the stages of Identity confusion and Identity comparison, due to the lack of awareness, acted in a way to protect the individuals emerging sexual orientation—'ignorance is bliss.' In these early stages, the individual has not started the process of revealing their orientation to others, and through using identity management and concealment (Cain, 1991), steer clear of hostility and constant worry.

Halpin and Allen (2004) believe the middle stages of orientation development are the most stressful for gays and lesbians. The researchers believe its during this time when individuals start to 'come out' to friends and family members, which could be followed by negative judgment, social stigma, decreased contact with others who are gay, a decrease in self-esteem and a lack of confidence in their emerging identity. The overall lifestyle change and different social interactions in adjusting to their new identity could be related to stress.

The ending stages of Identity pride and Identity synthesis are associated with a stable sexual identity and implies the presence of social relationships and support by significant others (Cass, 1979). The study by Halpin and Allen (2004) supports Cass' idea. The men at this stage of development report high self-esteem, increased satisfaction with life, are less lonely, and report being relatively happy. Cass (1979) believed that identity synthesis happens when the individual experiences a growing sense of harmony between the public and private self.

Finally, Halpin and Allen (2004) noted the average ages of the sample increased from Identity confusion through Identity synthesis, meaning a gay identity development occurs in stages in contrast to being a stable characteristic. Cass (1996) believes that individuals with negative attitudes towards their emerging orientation may have a different outlook when compared to those individuals with a positive attitude, which supports calls for a longitudinal study on orientation development.

Research by Savin-Williams (1995) looked at the relationships between pubertal maturation, sexual behavior, and self-esteem. One of the findings of the study was that same-sex sexual behavior followed the timing of maturation (i.e., early maturers started to have same-sex sexual encounter earlier than the later maturers) while sexual behavior with people of the opposite sex did not. So, for gay and bisexual youth, starting their same-sex sexual activity was correlated with biological cues, where sexual activity with the opposite sex started according to a social clock.

Earlier research on orientation was conducted by McDonald (1982), who studied 199 self-identifying gay males. Many of them reported a 'milestone event' in relation to accepting the sexual orientation. Some of these 'events' included (a) an awareness of a preference for same-sex relationship, (b) same-sex activity and experiences, (c) an understanding of term "homosexual," (d) a homosexual self-description, (e) the first homosexual relationship and (f) the adaptation of a positive gay identity. The McDonald study also found that gays recalled an awareness of same-sex attractions around 13 years old, with a same-sex experience and understanding the term "homosexual" occurring around 19 years old. The average age for first same-sex relationship occurring around 21 years old, while 'coming out' to a non-gay associate occurred around 23 years old. For many individuals in this study, they reported a positive gay identity was developed by 24 years old. {15% of the McDonald study did not see themselves as having a positive gay identity}.

In looking at lesbians, Minton and McDonald (1984) created a three-stage model for the development of a homosexual orientation. They believed the individual started at an *Egocentric* stage which appears in childhood or adolescence and involves genital contact, emotional attachment and fantasies about a member of one's own sex. The second stage is called *Sociocentric* where the individual internalized the negative social outlook of lesbians causing the person feel guilty and leading to secrecy and isolation. The final stage is called *Universalistic*, where she understands it is acceptable to questions social attitudes, accepts a positive homosexual identity and integrates the lesbian identity with other characteristics of herself.

Kitzinger and Wilkinson (1995) looked at women who were self-defined as heterosexual (for 10 years) and transitioned to lesbianism.

Reflecting the Minton and McDonald model, they also came up with a three stage model for a developing lesbian sexual orientation. Their stages were called Getting There, Making and Describing the Transition to Lesbian Identity and Going On.

In *Getting There*, these researchers believe this is the stage where women do much of the preparatory 'work' to create a context to create a new orientation while doing their best to avoid confronting the possibility of a lesbian identity. In asking herself if she was a lesbian, one woman said:

> "I had growing feeling that I wanted … well, I didn't know what I did want … I blocked it out; I never finished that sentence even in my own mind. Looking back, it's obvious that I wanted to know women closely and, clearly, sexually, but I couldn't and didn't believe it. It seemed too extraordinary, too way out, too unlike my life, which was a secure middle-class life with a husband and two children. There wasn't any room for my fantasies—I tucked them away and hid them even from myself" (p.98).

In this same stage, there are sub-stages as well. Kitzinger and Wilkinson noted women also went through areas they named "we're just good friends", "It's just sex—I was only experimenting," and believing that "She's lesbian, not me."

In the second stage *Marking and Describing the Transition to Lesbian Identity*, the woman has reached the point and is able to claim a lesbian identity. One of the key factors in this stage is there is an event described as an "essential awakening"—an instant of recognition, of naming herself as a lesbian. One woman recalled:

> "It was really a special moment. I was going out with this man and I was bored out of my head but I was lying to myself, trying to talk myself into liking him, into believing he was potentially quite a nice bloke. And my friend Karen said, "… but Pauline, you don't even sound as if you *like* him." And we'd talked before about how maybe I could be a lesbian, and she just looked at me

and said, "You *are!*" and I said "I *am!*" and we celebrated it, and I knew there was no going back" (p.100).

In their final stage of *Going On*, the individual continues to discover what being a lesbian means to her, how she will live her life as a lesbian, and what kind of lesbian she wants to be. To explain, she accepts herself as lesbian and she becomes more lesbian. A part of this growth involves recalling unrecognized feelings or forgotten experiences. For example, one woman recalled:

> "When that happened, I got in touch with my own background. And remembered that I had had these kinds of thoughts as a high-school kid, that I had crushed on women, that not only that, that I had had two small sexual experiences with women, and both were cases where I can touched their breasts. And that there was a period in my all-girls high school where I had worn men's shirts" (cited in Ponse, 1978 p.162).

In their study of documenting the transition from heterosexuality to lesbianism, Kitzinger and Wilkinson (1995) concluded their evidence does not fit into an essentialist's model of orientation development. They acknowledge the constructionist ideal of their model which aids in understanding the processes of self and identity acceptance. This is their account of how women transition and interpret their changing orientation in relation to their comprehension of the category lesbian.

A few researchers challenge the idea of a stable lesbian identity. According to Reynolds and Hanjorgiris (2000) and Rust (1992), they felt that becoming a lesbian is method of self-classification that highlights the flexibility of sexual orientation.

For example, Sophie (1986) developed a four-stage model for sexual identity development. There was a general consensus in the progress through the stages, particularly the early stages. As the researcher progress through the later stages, the flexibility of a lesbian orientation appeared when 3 of the 14 women reported a preference towards heterosexuality. Sophie noted, "… we are mistaken if we interpret the notion of stability to mean the individuals who have become lesbian cannot subsequently change …" (p.49).

Later, Chapman and Brannock (1987) studied 197 on their development of a lesbian identity. In contrast to the Sophie (1986) study, they concluded the women were <u>consistent</u> with a "proposed model of lesbian identity awareness and self-labeling" (p. 79). They noted some of the women in their sample reported early experiences of "feeling connected to other girls/women" which led to "incongruence,"—the awareness that a same-sex relationship is atypical from the heterosexual norm. Next, women then questioned and explored their feelings and later on, identified as lesbians. So, these women never wavered and ended up with a same-sex partner (or, remained single but maintained a lesbian sexual orientation).

Others believe that there are multiple development pathways that lead to parallel results (Diamond & Savin-Williams, 2000). Meaning, people who had vastly different upbringings could end up as colleagues at work. Thinking sexually, knowing how some individuals label their sexual identity does not actually tell us about their life experiences or the nature of their current erotic behavior (Peplau & Garnets, 2000).

Some of the newer ideas on the development of sexual orientation believe they are diverse and complex. For example, in contrast to step-by-step model, the development may be non-linear (Rust, 1996). Other scientists have challenged 'step' models. Research found that many people actually do not follow 'step' models (Diamond, 2000). Diamond (2000) looked at the sexual attractions, behaviors, and identities of gays and lesbians over a two-year period. 40% of the sample noted their sexual attraction varied and they did not assign the 'variation' to changes in awareness. Also, 50% of the young women in the study mentioned they had changed their 'identity label' more than once since dropping their heterosexual identity. This study displays one example of the personal process one goes through in arriving at a sexual identity.

Moving on, studies suggest that childhood behaviors and experiences are important factors due to the idea that sexual orientation exerts pressure on development before the appearance on same-sex attractions. Many adult gay men recalled as youths of having a sense of being different from others (Bell et al., 1981). These feelings may have appeared as self-perceptions of gender-atypicality, fascination with same-sex peers or adults, the sense that one does not want the other gender or one is unsure of what he or she actually wants (Savin-Williams, 1995). To add, many adult gay men remember engaging in gender-atypical behaviors during childhood (Bailey, 1996) while studies report that the frequency of extremely feminine boys who ultimately professed a homosexual orientation was higher than expected by chance (Green, 1987).

Other research found that the feelings of being "different" have a rather low correlation when compared to same-sex orientations among women as with men. The relationship is rather small (Bailey & Zucker, 1995). Lesbian women remembered more gender-atypical behaviors than both bisexual and heterosexual women (Philips & Over, 1995) but, there was substantial overlap among groups: Some lesbians remembered a feminine upbringing while some heterosexual women reported being tomboys. Further, some gay men reported gender-typical childhoods (Philips & Over, 1992) while some gender-atypical boys developed heterosexual orientations (Green, 1987). While the research suggest that the relationship between childhood gender atypically and adult sexual orientation is stronger among men than women, authors caution in understanding its significance for the development of female sexual orientation (Bailey, 1996).

When individuals reach adolescence, the sexual individual increases in importance and the issues for non-heterosexuals begin to appear (Boxer & Cohler, 1989). Due to persistent heterosexism of ones environment, talking about same-sex feelings can be dangerous so, feelings of isolation tend to dominate the questioning youth. D'Augelli (1989) found that college student recalled 'gaps' of years between their initial same-sex attractions and talking to another about those feeling. Those who dare to come out as gay or lesbian during the teen years are more likely to experience discrimination and violence, both at home and at school (D'Augelli, 1989). The possible results of this negative environment include feeling depressed and/or thoughts of or committing suicide (Savin-Williams, 1994). While the acceptance of a gay or lesbian identity is thought to occur during the teen years, some individuals may identity themselves as non-heterosexual for the first time after they have become adults (Brown, 1996).

For women, they usually experience their first homosexual attraction and begin questioning their sexual identity at a later age than males (Bell & Weinberg, 1978). Where questioning and bisexual men tend to focus on sexual attraction, women place a greater focus on their emotional feelings for the same sex (Blumstein & Schwartz, 1990). Also, some women begin to question their sexual identities for reasons that are not related to same-sex attractions which may include being exposed to ideological beliefs, gays and lesbians, and/or community events (Cass, 1990).

There may be other differences between lesbians and gay men (Garnets & Peplau, 2000). Studies suggest that patterns of sexual thoughts, behaviors, and attractions appear to be linked to gender but not to sexual orientation (Diamond, & Savin-Williams, 2000). Further, females tend to have relational or partnered-centered orientation to sexuality where males tend to focus on recreational or body-centered orientations (Baldwin & Baldwin, 1997). To explain, Regan and Berscheid (1996) asked "what is sexual desire?" A couple of the responses were:

> Male: Sexual desire is wanting someone ... in a physical manner. No strings attached. Just uninhibited sexual intercourse.
> Female: Sexual desire is the longing to be emotionally intimate and to express love for another person.

Also, both heterosexuals and homosexual males report more sex partners than females (Bell & Weinberg, 1978). In 1987, Paroski found that 95% of gay men and only 16% of lesbians learned about homosexuality through sexual encounters. In the same study, 81% of male and 31% of females went to locations thought or known to be gay or lesbian. So, it was concluded that gender seems to be stronger than sexual orientation in affecting male and female sexuality.

Other gender differences have appeared as well. Various studies have found that homosexual women report higher rates of prior heterosexual activity versus homosexual males (Savin-Williams, 1990). While these behaviors may not indicate lesbians are more interested in heterosexual activity, Weinberg et al. (1994) proposed that social pressure may make it more difficult for women than men to avoid heterosexual sexual activity.

Nature or Nurture?

To begin the discussion on the "cause" of homosexuality, it is important to look at this issue from a number of perspectives. To start with the scientific perspective which is said to be 'value-free', which seeks to explore and increase our knowledge about the world around us. The immediate significance of findings are often unclear and their eventual consequences are unpredictable (Marmor, 1998).

From an ethical standpoint, the "cause" of homosexuality should not be important at all. The ethical issue of most importance should be if ones behavior is dangerous or destructive to others. Marmor (1998) says:

> "Whether homosexuality is innate, acquired, consciously chosen, or any combination of these, the highest ethical imperative in a humanistic society mandates that gays and lesbians be treated no differently than any other religious, ethnic, or racial group, or indeed, than heterosexuals in general." (p.20)

Finally, looking at homosexuality from a socio-politico-religious perspective, the issue of "cause" gains in importance due to prejudice and hostility directed towards them. Like prejudice and hostility found in other areas of life, homophobia is based on the lack of knowledge about gays and lesbians. Socially based homophobia is commonly based on at least four assumptions: (1) it is sinful—the idea that is mainly supported on religious ground; (2) it is an unnatural behavior—supported by teleological assumptions on the reproduction of the species; (3) homosexuality is a 'chosen' behavior and can be 'un-chosen'; and (4) that is potentially contagious and one can be 'infected' by social exposure (Marmor, 1989).

Some of the other ideas on the cause of homosexuality include the idea that gays hate or fear women due to negative feelings towards their mother. In contrast, another idea is that gays strongly identify with their mothers therefore, their attraction to other men appears. A third idea on the cause of homosexuality is that homosexual behavior is caused by pre-oedipal issues with separation and individuation from the mother (Socarides, 1968).

One of the more popular psychoanalytic ideas on the cause of homosexuality is the close-binding, seductive mother and distant, unloving father (Bieber et al., 1962). This family set-up has been considered that source of castration anxieties, the fear/hate of women, and the feminine identifications seen in gays. Siegelman (1974) demonstrated such a family set-up has appeared in the histories of heterosexual men which did not lead to homosexual behaviors. Further, gays and lesbians have been found to come from quite a varied background. Studies found over 50 variables/family patterns in the histories of homosexuals: loving mothers, hostile mothers, loving fathers, hostile fathers, idealized fathers, sibling rivalries; intact homes, broken homes, absent mothers, absent fathers, etc (Hatterer, 1970). Bieber et al. (1962) concluded that the idea of a loving father prevents the development of a gay son is not true. To add, later research found that 17% of gays in a sample felt themselves to be their father's favorite (Bell, Weinberg, & Hammersmith, 1981).

One of the major categories in the discussion around the 'cause' of homosexuality is known as essentialism. Experts tend to agree the concept of essentialism originated in the work of Plato (Mayr, 1982) but it was later defined by Irvine (1990) as the belief that certain phenomena are natural, inevitable, universal, and biologically determined. Researchers use biological evidence to support their idea that there is a biologic cause for homosexuality.

Researchers have looked at monozygotic (MZ) twins and dizygotic (DZ) twins (Bailey & Pillard, 1991; Whitam et al., 1993) which revealed some possible correlations for homosexuality, (52% to 22%) among MZ twins compared to the DZ twins. A trait that is genetically-based should display itself identically in MZ twins—they are clones. DZ (fraternal) twins are no more related than non-twin brother. Further, the Whitam research included a set of MZ triplets were all three were homosexual. Scientists say findings like these do not represent a genetic 'cause' for homosexuality but, they accept the chance of genetic factor that aids in homosexual development.

Whitam et al (1993) published work on male twins that shows a higher occurrence of homosexuality in MZ twins. The research mentions two gay twins who were unknown to each other, living in different cities where both of them photographed shirtless construction workers over the age of 40 and later at home masturbated to the photographs.

In talking about a possible genetic 'cause', it is important to mention the work of Dean Hamer et al. (1993). Hamer researched 40 families with two homosexual brothers. Hamer took blood samples from gay brothers and the mother and compared X-chromosome sequences looking for a sting of genetic material shared by both gay brothers. Hamer observed that the Xq28 region of the X-chromosome was shared by 33 of the 40 gay brothers. It needs to be said that this region of the X-chromosome contains several hundred genes so it is a bit premature to declare the discovery of the gay gene.

Other researchers have focused on hormonal differences between homosexuals and heterosexual to aid in finding a cause of homosexuality. Kolodny et al (1971) found that homosexual men had lower levels of circulating testosterone than heterosexual men. To add, the Kolodny group found that circulating testosterone levels dropped significantly along the Kinsey Scale from exclusively heterosexual through bisexual to exclusively homosexual men. Later information from the Kolodny (1972) data found high levels of circulating luteinizing hormone (LH). Dorner et al. (1975) gave injections of estrogens to gay males and noted that LH in this sample followed a response pattern that was more typical of females than males. There was an early decrease in the LH level followed by a positive rebound above the baseline, where the group of heterosexual males did not show the same type of rebound. Almost 20 years later, the Dorner group (1991) proposed that high adrenal androgens during the prenatal period of brain organization result in an increased chance for one to become bisexual or homosexual, with a greater chance in female and a slightly lesser chance in males. Dorner's idea is that high levels of androgenic steroids lead to male-typical gender behaviors and homosexuality in women and decreased testicular androgens aid in the creation of a homosexual disposition in males. Glaude et al (1984) also did work looking at LH and homosexuals. In their research, they found that the physiological response to a LH injection revealed a stable pattern level that fell between heterosexual males and females. Research like these point to the possibility of the hypothalamic area having been androgenized compared to heterosexual males.

Also of interest, women with pregnancy issues were given large doses of diethylstilbestrol (DES), a synthetic estrogen, in the 1950s and 1960s. Since then, their children have been studied to see if prenatal exposure affected their sexuality. Since DES is an estrogen, the majority of concern was focused on the males but it was the females who showed sexual effects. Mayer-Bahlburg et al. (1995) found less than half of the DES women had a bias towards bisexuality or homosexuality. The men who were exposed to DES were more likely to report depressive disorders (Pillard, 1993).

Moving into the brain, there has been neuranatomic evidence for the cause of homosexuality. For example, LeVey (1991) found that the third interstitial nucleus of the anterior hypothalamus (INAH-3) was distinctly smaller (less than half the size) in homosexual males as compared to heterosexual males. Published a year earlier, Swaab and

Hofman (1990) were looking at the brains if patients with a dementing illness such as Alzheimer's disease. They noticed that the suprachiasmatic nucleus (SCN—it aids in the coordination of the biorhythms of the body) showed cell loss and reduced volume. They wondered in the same would appear in patients with AIDS dementia. They compared non-demented homosexual men with AIDS *to* heterosexual men with AIDS *to* heterosexual men dying of other diseases. They found larger SCN's, with twice as many cells, in the homosexual sample.

Laura Allen and Roger Gorski (1992) looked at the anterior commissure (AC) in 34 homosexual men, 75 heterosexual men and 84 heterosexual women. The AC houses connecting neurons for both sides of the brain which allows the transfer of information. They found that the anterior commissure was significantly larger in homosexual men than heterosexual men or women. Other research found that gays and lesbians differ from heterosexuals on some cognitive abilities, although the differences have been small (Glaude & Bailey, 1995).

Other researchers support the idea of social influence on an individual's experience. This is known as <u>Social Constructionism</u> where the basic idea of the paradigm is that reality is socially constructed (Berger & Luckmann, 1966). Berger and Luckmann (1966) accept that idea that sexuality is based on biological drives. They argue that biology does not determine where, when and with what a person engages in sexual behavior. They said:

> "Sexuality ... [is] channeled in specific directions socially rather than biologically, a channeling that not only imposes limits on these activities, but directly affects organismic functions" (p.181).

A few years later, Simon and Gagnon's book *Sexual Conduct* (1973) developed an idea where sexuality is primarily socially constructed. They rejected the essentialist's notion of biology and later, Gagnon (1990) argued that "sexuality is not ... [a] universal phenomenon which is the same in all historical time and cultural spaces" (p.3). The culture creates sexuality by defining behaviors which teaches members of this society through social scripts.

Aside from biology, genes and hormones, social constructionists support the idea of variations across cultures in the behaviors associated with homosexuality and heterosexuality. Blackwood (1993) concluded from anthropological data that:

> "Patterns of homosexual behavior reflect the value systems and social structure of the different societies in which they are found. The ideology regarding male and female roles, kinship and marriage regulation, and the sexual division of labor are all important in the construction of homosexual behavior" (p.331).

Further, there can be various forms of sexual behavior with in a lifestyle. Broad and overreaching comparisons between homosexual and heterosexual men miss the many forms of behaviors. There are celibate and devoted gay men while there are married heterosexual men with a high number of extra-marital sex partners. This wide range of variability is inconsistent with essentialist concepts (Fausto-Sterling, 1986).

To end this discussion on Social Constructionism, many essentialists support the idea of sexual constancy over the lifetime of the individual—one is heterosexual or homosexual for life. Yes, there are societies where sexual orientation appears fixed throughout the lifespan. In contrast, there are other societies were sexual orientations vary during the lifespan (DeLamater & Shibley-Hyde, 1998). There is the well documented case of the Sambia reported by Herdt (1984). The male youth engage in primarily homosexual behaviors. Following marriage, they continue homosexual behaviors with youth and heterosexual behaviors with their wife. Following the birth of their first child, the males become exclusively heterosexual.

My Study/Conclusion

Well, after reading and writing about all of the various methods for defining, measuring and the etiology of homosexuality, I have come to the conclusion that this is a worthless line of research. Where it is universally understood that fire will burn, sexual orientation varies within societies and cultures. All cultures understand that fire burns and gives off heat where not all cultures and societies universally condemn same-sex orientations and behaviors. I believe there are so many other area of research where sexual scientists could better spend their time. Trying to define homosexuality is a useless endeavor. It's like catching the wind in your hand. When you think you have it, it just blows away. There are so many variations, why even bother to try and just let people be. Secondly, why are people looking for a 'cause' of homosexuality? Luckily, few or none of the studies on genes have been replicated. For me, when I hear 'cause', I also look at the other side: cure. Hey, while they are looking for things, why not look for a cure for Blackness or left-handedness. But, since it was apart of the assignment, I'll answer the questions you provided.

Question. For my study, I would like to see if I could determine if homosexuality was a choice in the Black male college population. There seems to be an awful lot of discussion about men on the "DL." I would avoid the discussion on HIV/STD transmission in this community since men on the DL are being blamed for the spread of HIV to 'heterosexual' Black women.

Measure. (Please keep in mind my previous statements about measuring orientations). I would use an idea similar to Shively and DeCecco (1977) of putting heterosexuality and homosexuality on separate scales. Like some of the other researchers, I believe putting making homosexuality and heterosexual polar opposites (i.e. Kinsey Scale) is the wrong thing to do. I would ask my sample (1) what they felt their sexual identity to be (heterosexual, bisexual, homosexual, other, etc.) and (2) what would significant others (family, friends) assume the individuals' sexual orientation to be. Then, I would ask them to note the frequency of their (3) sexual behaviors on a heterosexual or homosexual scale—their choice! Some individuals many respond on the heterosexual scale, homosexual scale or both scales. Finally, I would ask them to comment on the frequency of (4) sexual fantasies—homosexual or heterosexual—their choice. I believe the most important information is what they define themselves to be in relation to their choice of scale on the behavior and fantasy scale.

Sample. Well, in order to gather a fairly large sample, I would visit historically Black colleges and universities (HBCU's). I would include colleges such as Hampton and Norfolk State in Virginia, Delaware State in Delaware, and Cheney University and Lincoln University located in Pennsylvania. I would like to link up with some of the professors from these schools and use some of their classes in my sample. With luck, a large sample would decrease the sample bias error.

Data. For starters, I would use a survey to gather the information. No experiments or anything like that. For starters, I would get basic demographic information (age, grade level, race, etc). {The reason I would gather race is because some professors would allow those students who took part in the study to have extra credit for a test or something. It would be unfair to only allow the Black students to have access to the extra points}. I would like to use 2 separate tools. First I would like to use a basic survey that looked measured ones orientation with my two-tiered approach to measuring orientation attached to the end. Secondly, I would like to use some sort of measurement tool that looked at what the individual thought his/her friends though their orientation to be. {I don't know if I said that right}. This tool would look at perceptions of being true to oneself and openness or 'out-ness.'

Analysis. For the analysis of this research, I would use a t-test to look for the means of each score on the survey. Then, I would take the mean scores and compare them to the self-identity tool to see if there was a weak/strong correlation between an individual's orientation and their self-identity. Finally, I would take the mean scores from the orientation survey and compare them to the scores from the friends' perception of orientation scale to see look acceptance and openness regarding the individual's orientation and identity.

Strengths. Well, it is kind of tough to try and support a research topic that I disagree with. I can say that my sample is generalizable to Black college males. Thinking nationally, that is a rather small number of individuals so I do believe the generalizabilty should be fairly high. Secondly, I would gather my sample from various regions around the country, not just one unique college or university to aid with generalizability. Third, I do believe this is a new area of research so, just looking at this topic broadens the knowledge of sexuality.

Weaknesses. To end this essay, I can say one of the major issues with this research would be the lack of enthusiasm for this topic. Secondly, in trying to create a definition for an individual's orientation, I am sure there will be some who feel they are not represented by the measurement tool. Third, since being on the 'DL' is problematic enough and even with the promise on anonymity, I do not believe some of the males would be honest regarding their sexual behaviors.

7

Theory of Reasoned Action

Research presented by the Centers for Disease Control has shown a gradual increase in HIV infections contracted through heterosexual intercourse (Centers for Disease Control, 1994). At the same time, other research found that most heterosexuals continue to believe themselves not to be at risk for HIV infection and have not changed their sexual behavior. One national survey found that less than one-fifth of heterosexuals with an HIV risk factor reported consistenly using condoms (Catania et al., 1992). These statistics suggests that health-education messages directed at the general population have not had the intended effect. Warning the public and offering facts about HIV transmission may be an important factor in behavior change. But, it is unlikely these messages by themselves are enough to change ingrained sexual habits, expectations, and attitudes that are often supported by the values and norms of the dominant culture or particular subcultures. A major step in creating more effective prevention and behavior-change programs is to understand the social-psychological determinants of people's decision to adopt AIDS risk-reducing behaviors (Wulfert & Wan, 1995).

Despite widespread awareness of the risks involved, risky behavior (unprotected intercourse) remains common, and preventive behavior (using condoms) remain inconsistent among gay men (Kelly et al., 1990) minorities, and heterosexually active people in general (Catania et al., 1992). People identified as being a part of a risk group are likely to have more than one sexual partner and display an inconstant use of condoms (Moore & Rosenthal, 1991). Even though research has found an acceptable level of HIV knowledge in these groups, there is a discrepancy between their knowledge and beliefs about HIV prevention and the actual safety of their own sexual behavior (Turtle et al, 1989).

Additional research by Emmons (et al., 1986) found several factors that were related to 'change' in order to avoid risk. These factors included knowledge regarding AIDS, perceived risk of AIDS, and the perceived efficacy of behavior change for reducing one's chances of developing AIDS. Other factors related only to behaviors that would alter the number or type of one's sexual partner included difficulties with sexual impulses, belief in biomedical technology to prevent/cure AIDS, and perceived social norms.

Baldwin and Baldwin (1988) looked at various cognitive-emotional variables, including individuals' knowledge about AIDS, perceived risk, and personal concern about "cautions behavior." The researchers defined 'cautions behavior' in terms of condom use, a low number of sexual partners, and participation in casual sex. They found that none of these variables mentioned had much influence on "cautions behavior."

Finally, Walter (et. al., 1992) looked at students living in an AIDS epicenter. They found that students who perceived group norms inconsistent with AIDS preventive behaviors (i.e. friends who had intercourse never or inconsistently used condoms, etc.) were more likely to indicate they had engaged in riskier AIDS related behavior.

Researchers have been trying to understand AIDS risk and AIDS-preventive behavior since the beginning of the AIDS epidemic, while the application of formal theory in this area has been relatively rare (Coates, 1990). This unsystematic approach to researching AIDS risk and AIDS prevention has resulted in the accumulation of unrelated findings concerning variables that affect AIDS risk and AIDS prevention. The potential for theory-driven research has been largely unrealized (Fisher & Fisher, 1992).

TRA

The Theory of Reasoned Action (TRA) (Ajzen & Fishbein, 1980; Fishbein & Ajzen, 1975) is a cognitive model, where the application of the theory has provided strong and valid predictions of a variety of health-related decisions including decisions about abortion (Smetana & Adler, 1980), birth planning intentions (Crawford & Boyer, 1985), intentions to use drugs (Bentler & Speckart, 1979), and contraceptive decision making (Davidson & Morrison, 1983).

The TRA suggests that a person's intention to perform a specific behavior is a function of his or her affective response to performing the behavior (attitudes) and perceived social norms about the behavior. Attitudes are predicted by the person's beliefs about the likelihood and evaluation of the consequences of performing the behavior (outcome beliefs). Perceived social norms are based on the person's beliefs regarding the wishes regarding specific relevant beliefs and his or her desire to conform to those norms (normative beliefs) (Baker, Morrison, Carter & Verdon, 1996).

Stated another way, an individuals AIDS-preventive behavior is a function of her or his behavioral intentions to perform a particular preventive act. Behavior intentions are assumed to be a function of the individual's attitude toward performance of a particular preventive behavior, the individual's subjective norm or perception of what significant others wish the individual to do with respect to the behavior in question, or both (Ajzen & Fishbein, 1980; Fishbein & Ajzen, 1975).

In relation to AIDS/HIV prevention, a person's attitude toward the performance of a particular AIDS preventative behavior is a function of the person's beliefs about the consequences of performing the behavior, multiplied by his or her evaluation of these consequences. At the same time, this theory holds that an individual's subjective norm is a function of his or her perception of social support from specific "others" in the performance of the preventive behavior, multiplied by his or her motivation to comply with these "others" individuals' wishes (Fisher, Fisher & Rye, 1995). The TRA proposes that is important to conduct research to identify beliefs about the consequences of preventive behaviors, and sources of social influence (referents) for preventive behavior, that are important for the particular population and for preventative behavior of interest, rather than arrive at these beliefs and referents through trial and error (Ajzen & Fishbein, 1980).

The overall strength of the TRA appears in its definition of variables the statement of the relationship between variables. The individual's *attitude toward the behavior* and *perceptions of social norms* regarding the behavior are sufficient for predicting intention to perform that behavior. Other variables are believed to work through their influence on these two main variables (Baker, Morrison, Carter & Verdon, 1996).

Moving On ...

One study found no correlation between knowledge of AIDS and sexual behavior which suggests that a strictly information-only program to AIDS prevention education will not be very effective. This finding was supported by other research. Baum and Nesselhof (1988) stated that the "Social influence variables and personality may also affect the decision to engage in risky behavior and may determine the appropriateness and effectiveness of educational campaigns and other preventive efforts" (p.905). Also, the findings from this research regarding perceived peer norms may imply if AIDS education is to be effective, it must penetrate the culture. In other words, practicing safer sex must somehow become the group norm, which does not seem to be the case today (Winslow, Franzini & Hwang, 1992).

For many years, the prevailing preventive model was informational health messages presented by the media and in the classroom (Calamidas, 1990). There is evidence that the strictly informational approach is not sufficient to induce behavior change. "Information is a necessary but insufficient condition for behavior change: belief in one's vulnerability and in the severity of consequences of HIV disease, as well as, some prompt or stimulus to change the behavior is necessary" (O'Keefe, Nasselhof-Kendall & Baum, 1990, p.170). It has been suggested that these "beliefs" are changed by using group or normative pressures. Research has found that the peer-based education was an aid for changing group beliefs. The use of peers led to significant improvements among participants' knowledge, attitudes, and behavior intentions (Shulkin et al., 1991).

Modeling the decision to use condoms to use condoms provided useful information for the design of education programs to specific groups. Research found with steady partners, the attitude toward the behavior and perceived social norm regarding the behavior were related to the intention to use condoms. Therefore, these results suggest that safer sex programs focused on increasing condom usage with steady partners should be directed to the members of the sexual relationship. In other words, to motivate condom usage with steady partners, it is necessary to influence the attitudes and norms of both partners (Baker, Morrison, Carter & Verdon, 1996).

Research has found that women are more likely to respond to education programs that emphasize normative influences such as program designed to change perceived social norms for condom use or education programs designed to teach women to counter and change their partner's negative responses to condoms. In contrast, men were found to respond to educational programs designed to change their own attitudes. Research also found, among men and women, those who were more familiar with condoms (through prior use), were more likely to intend to use them. Therefore, prevention program should give participants the chance to see and handle condoms and develop the skills in both negotiating use and the actual mechanics of use (Baker, Morrison, Carter & Verdon, 1996).

It was also suggested that looking at specific outcomes and normative beliefs underlying attitudes and norms also provides assistance when designing prevention education programs. The bonus of looking at the relationship of beliefs to intentions appears when, for example, looking at the beliefs about the effectiveness of condoms for preventing STD's. Most participants believe that condoms are effective for preventing STD's. At the same time, while this belief is important to an individual's attitude towards condoms, it is not related to their intention to use condoms (Baker, Morrison, Carter & Verdon, 1996). To add, when designing programs, looking at the beliefs that distinguish between those who do and do not intend to use condoms due to issues of sexual pleasure, interrupting sex, and access to condoms is also important. Research found that subjects who intend to use condoms, with steady or casual partners, perceive that their partner think they should use them. Both men and women perceive that their steady partners are less likely to favor condoms than their casual partners, and are more motivated to comply with steady partners than with casual partners (Baker, Morrison, Carter & Verdon, 1996).

As Teaching Tool?

Safer-sex interventions with heterosexual populations that have focused on AIDS/HIV education have not uniformly encouraged safer sexual behavior (Fisher & Fisher, 1992). The overall lack of reliable success may be due in part to perceived invulnerability to HIV/ AIDS among heterosexuals, although specifics of design and interventions may have also affected desired outcomes (Bryan, Aiken & West, 1996).

Due to the high intercorrelations among attitudes, norms, and self-efficacy, when creating educational interventions, it will be difficult to determine which variable is the most important or which precedes the other. Other evidence in other 'risk behaviors' suggests that educational interventions can influence changes in attitudes, norms, and self-efficacy which, in turn leads to changes in safer sex behavior (Holroyd, Penzien & Hursey, 1984).

When looking at variables that are related to behavior, it seems that factors to stress in education interventions may differ depending on the objective. For example, if the objective of sexuality education is to limit the number of sexual partners a person has, attitudes about having sexual intercourse would be an important factor to influence.

When using the TRA to reach this goal, an important part of the educational process would be to study the beliefs about the perceived consequences of having or abstaining from sexual intercourse and the evaluation of those consequences (Basen-Engquist & Parcel, 1992).

If the educational objective was to increase condom usage, influencing self-efficacy should be a major focus in the message. According to Bandura (1986), self-efficacy can be affected in four ways: (1) through mastery experiences or successful completion of the task, (2) role modeling or watching others perform the task (e.g. having peer educators demonstrate how to put a condom on a model), (3) social persuasion or information that the person can perform the task successfully, and (4) feedback on the physiological arousal states that help people infer their vulnerability to stress and anxiety. To increase self—efficacy regarding condom use, individuals need encouragement and successful experience with each of the steps involved in the behavior: (1) buying condoms, (2) taking them along on a date, (3) negotiating their use, and (4) putting them on (Basen-Engquist, Parcel, 1992).

Even though the TRA was created to predict and not necessarily change behaviors, educators have successfully used components of the TRA to guide the design of workshops that have increased male condom use (Kelly et al., 1991). One study found using the TRA to aid in program design was helpful but the research also revealed that interventions should be gender specific (Bogart, Cecil & Pinkerton, 2000).

For women, safer sex education programs should focus on changing social norms in favor of condom use, as well as, reducing negative attitudes towards condom use. In changing social norms, there have been safer sex programs which used popular members of the community to endorse and recommend safer sex behaviors to other members of their community. To add, research found that women who received factual information promoting condom usage, along with guided instructions for proper condom usage, were significantly more likely to at least try to incorporate safer-sex into their sexual behaviors than were women who did receive any education (Perry et al., 1996).

When looking at men, the same research stated their educations programs should focus on teaching them to negotiate condom use with potential sex partners (who do not like condoms) and to communicate their safer sex concerns to their partners (Bogart, Cecil & Pinkerton, 2000).

Future

The early education programs created to prevent HIV infection were not envisioned by theoretical models or research data to determine antecedents of risk behaviors. Overtime, programs appeared that were focused on theory which provided a better understanding of the underlying psychological variables that lead to risky behaviors.

Eventhough the findings of research support the ideas that self-efficacy and variables from the TRA are related with HIV-related sexual behavior, more research is need to develop better education models that are related to the variables that influence individuals' sexual behaviors. For example, it has been suggested that a more effective education program could be created by merging the TRA with the Social Learning Theory's variable of *outcome expectation* (the perception that performing the behavior would achieve the desires outcome). It is believed that such an approach would provide a more complete picture of the cognitive and social factors affecting an individuals' sexual behavior (Basen-Engquist & Parcel, 1992).

My Thoughts

As I was writing this little paper, I realized something. I thought back to 625 (an old class), when I told you I used the TRA and Trans-theoretical model. I realized I did not explain the TRA as well as I should. Actually, I explained the TRA in relation to myself and how I 'understood' (read: used) the theory. But at the same time, I was successful in getting people to practice safer sex and change their overall behaviors in order to decrease their risky behaviors.

For starters, I knew I was not the first person to talk to my group participants about practicing safer sex and I realized (without a scientific study) that just giving people information did not work, especially in the area of behavior change. Since HIV first appeared, educators have been singing the same song about condoms and safer sex. If those messages worked, the infection rate would have peaked in the 80's and should be near zero now. Well ... that did not work. The people in my groups needed something more.

Then, in the process of writing a continuation grant for my old job, I came across the TRA. Overtime, I figured out how to use it. For starters, I made myself the 'person in the community who endorsed safer sex'. By community, I mean my group presentations. I would see the same group for a period of 2 months. Overall, the groups liked me and they respected my information and opinions (how I did that, I have no clue). I like to think I created an environment where it was ok for people to talk about their fears and about not getting the virus. At the same time, my groups knew I was pro-sex and I did my best to educate them on other areas of their sexuality, not just HIV. In other words, I created my own little safer sex bubble, my own *community norms*.

In the groups, I did my best to change people *attitudes* in regards to condoms and safer sex. I stressed the fact it was a good idea to use condoms. Since I was the 'respected member', I said to many of my groups "Hey ... I don't like to use condoms either but, I know the consequences so, I use Crown condoms." I told them the specific brand that I used and I also passed them out to the participants so they could try them. I would say something like "yall know me, and I like to get my freak on, and I never had a Crown condom break on me." I would also say to the guys that "they are so thin, you can't even tell that you're wearing one." So, it was my hope their brain processes went something like '... ya know, if he uses these condoms and swears by them, they can't be that bad because he's a sex expert.'

Also, I would tell my groups about alternatives to intercourse. For example, I would give out flavored condoms and flavored dental damns. I remember we were discussing using a flavored condoms for oral sex. One woman said 'she wanted to try flavored condoms but her johns did not like them.' So, another woman taught her, in class, how to put on a condom with her mouth. I had a dildo with me and she practiced in class. Within five minutes, she was a pro. (I just like to tell that story).

Anyhow, I tried my best to get my groups to realize it was in their overall best interest not to get infected. I guess you could call that an *outcome*. I believe self-efficacy was high because we practiced safer behaviors in class, including negotiating safer sex and how to use condoms. I also believe the use of peers (people who were their age & similar life circumstances but, with HIV). The peers explained how they were infected and the impact it had on their families. The peers also mentioned the monetary aspect to having the virus. The peers constantly mentioned the red-tape they went through in order to get government assistance or pay the $1500+ per month in medication. Usually, the peers would end their time talking about feeling sick—having good days and bad days. To end ... I think the combination of the techniques came together in a way to get people to learn about HIV and ways to avoid infection.

How did I measure success? A minor goal was to get the guys in the group to stop carrying their condoms in their wallet, due to the heat damaging the latex. I had several guys go out of their way to show me they were now carrying their condoms in the inside jacket packet. That may seem like a minor victory but in HIV prevention education, you take what you can get.

Secondly, the guys would come back to me and ask for the Crown condoms by name. Granted, I had other brands of condoms with me, my guys would say something like 'Yeah man.... I used those condoms you gave me over the weekend and they were "da bomb" ... umm ... do you have any more of those Crowns?' I also noticed this with the flavored condoms. The women in the group said they liked the taste while, the guys responded to how their girlfriends responded to the taste (meaning, their girlfriend's liked the taste and therefore, were more "aggressive" when performing oral sex).

I really do not know what else to say. I can say from my own experience, using the TRA in combination with other teaching strategies (peers, role play, hands-on demonstrations, etc.) led to behavior change for participants in my group. No, I was able to help everyone but I know in needed more time in order to reach them.

8

Sex Can Wait, Damn It!

The topic of this article is about abstinence-only sex education. We will briefly go through the resent research regarding STI's and out of wedlock births. Then we will go discuss the recent change in government involvement where abstinence only education has been brought back to the forefront where it belongs. We will end with an evaluation of several abstinence-only programs that were well received by the students as well as the teachers. Those people who have promoted sexuality education for our children have done them a great disservice and it needs to be corrected. Instead of allowing condoms to be distributed in our classroom, the children need to receive an entirely different message. The children should be told to wait until marriage before they begin sexual activity.

American schools and what behaviors take place in them are changing. Violence, alcohol and drugs, sexual behavior, and family values are concerns for parents, teachers, and students now more than ever. Think about some of the following facts:

- Homicide rates in the United States are more than twice as high as in other industrialized country (Butterfield, 1992).

- Concerns about young people's use of alcohol, marijuana, and other relatively mild drugs is rising because it reflects an overall alienation from social values that many believe are critical to successful transition to adulthood (Ornstein & Levine, 1993).

• Although the number of births among teenagers fell substantially during the 1970's and early 1980's the birth rate per 1,000 women 15-19 years of age has increased, and the percentage of out-of-wedlock births to teenagers has increased substantially from 15% in 1960 to nearly 75% in 1991 (Ornstein & Levine, 1993).

• School administrators and teachers are facing increased public pressure to respond to the AIDS pandemic with increased and effective risk-reduction education for all children; at the same time, many parents and educators are incensed by programs involving distribution of condoms in big-city schools (Altman, 1991, Ornstein & Levine, 1993).

Remaining abstinent during the adolescent years may be one of the toughest challenges facing our youth today. The number of sexual messages our children receive by way of the print and mass media each day makes it increasingly tough to maintain their virgin status. During the 1960, adolescent issues dealt with on television were rather innocuous and included dates, blemishes, after-school jobs, and cars. During the 1990's adolescent issues portrayed on television included suicide, pregnancy, HIV/AIDS, sexual harassment and sexual abuse (Perry, Kelder, and Kormro, 1993). It was also observed that the ratio of heterosexual unmarried to married couples was 24 to 1, reinforcing the message that sexual behavior is more likely to occur outside of marriage (Lowry & Towles, 1989a). Lowry and Towles (1989b) also found that children watch 11 sexual behaviors per hour during prime time television. Add the impact of films, music video's, and the world wide web and it become evident that the children in the United States today learn about sex through an almost unlimited exposure to sexual scenes where protection and responsibility are absent (Perry, Kelder, and Kormro, 1993).

Sexual intercourse adds to many health and social problems for the children of the United States. The birth rate of our children have actually dropped during the past few years, but the number of teenage pregnancies has remained constant at about 1 million per year (Ventura, Martin, Mathews & Clarke, 1996). Among our children, sexually transmitted disease, including Chlamydia, syphilis and human papillomavirus (HPV), are still widespread: one in seven children aged 15-19 contract a STD annually (CDC, 1997). By 1996, among 13 to 19 year olds, there were 2,574 reported AIDS cases and 3,041 other children known to be infected with HIV. Among 20-24 year olds, there were 19,997 AIDS cases and 11,818 others known to be HIV-positive, most of whom were probably contracted HIV when they were teenagers (CDC, 1996).

Controversy continues to exist over school based sexuality education, despite the fact the sex education is suggested or mandated by 48 states (SIECUS, 1992). One study found many states that mandated sex education also mandated that programs provided by schools emphasize sexual abstinence (Kirby & scales, 1981).

A number of negative consequences are often associated with teenage sexual intercourse (Brindis, 1990). The younger the child when they become sexually active, the greater the likelihood that the youth would experience negative consequences. The degree of these negative consequences is potentially greater for younger children (Olsen, Wallace & Miller, 1984). Therefore, the legitimate goal of sexuality education is to postpone early sexual involvement. The research says that "value free" sexuality education programs (those that do not teach morality, i.e., abstinence) "have failed to prevent unplanned pregnancies (Khouzam, 1995)." One health educator who works in McLennan County Texas tells his students in his class that "virginity is a gift you get to give away only once in your life, and I hope you save it for marriage" (Morse, 1999).

According to science, the country is being led to believe condoms are safe at preventing HIV transmission. This may not be the case. In the videotape *Teen and Chastity: A Talk with Molly Kelly* (1988), Kelly states that condoms have a 10% failure rate for pregnancy and a 17% failure rate for preventing HIV transmission because HIV is 500 times smaller than sperm. Also, in The Pro-Life Activist's Encyclopedia, it is reported that condoms allow HIV to pass through because condom pores are 5 microns in size, while HIV is 0.1 Micron

(Clowes, 1994). The Encyclopedia also sites a study that found sero-conversion in 17% of women whose HIV-positive husbands "faithfully" used condoms (New York State catholic Bishops, 1993). Robert Rector, a research fellow at the Heritage Foundation who help to write the original abstinence-only education bill says "the programs simply tell them (the student) the more sex they have outside of marriage, the less will be their prospects for human happiness (Morse, 1999)."

Opponents of abstinence-only education call it "erotophobic" and fear it could prevent kids from learning what they need to know about sex. Others are saying abstinence-only programs could undo a decade of progress in education about safe sex. "Denying them information about contraception and STD protection puts them at risk," says Debra Haffner, former president of SEICUS. Pam Smallwood of Planned Parenthood says, "If all kids learn about sex is that if you touch it you'll die, how can you ever expect them to develop healthy relationships? (Morse, 1999)"

It is no surprise that sex-education technocrats consider parents and other laymen little more than obstacles to be overcome; concerned citizens have even forced changes to CDC curricula. Outraged parents in a town in California revolted against lesson plans that asked teachers to match same-sex students in sexual role-playing exercises. The lesson plan encouraged the pairing of Bob and Bill in a scene of sexual tension. After the change, Bob and Bill are now played by Lee and Chris (Mindus, 2000).

Some educators and policy makers are embracing a more comprehensive sex education. Waco (Texas) public schools declined federal and state grant money and opted instead for a curriculum that includes information about contraceptives. And in Missouri and California, new laws require sex education to be "medically accurate" in portraying the effectiveness of contraceptives (Morse, 1999).

Even government officials cannot support the use of condoms. Dr. William Archer, the former Deputy Secretary of Health and Human Services was quoted saying "One out of three sexually active teenagers will acquire an STD before graduating from high school. And in most cases, a condom would have done little to stop it" (Griffin, 1993). Some of the abstinence-only programs may vary, but the federally funded programs require that children be taught the "harmful psychological and physical effects" of premarital sex. Former governor of Texas George W. Bush poured 6 million into the Texas abstinence-only education program. During several of President Bush's campaign stops, he pledged he would allocate $135 million dollars, or the amount the government spends on contraceptive programs, to "elevate abstinence education from an afterthought to an urgent priority. (Morse, 1999, p. 79)"

A youth services program at Atlanta's Grady memorial Hospital found that of the girls under age 16, 9 out of 10 wanted to learn how to say no. One way to teach them is for adults to teach them reasons to say no and give them the moral support to keep saying no (Bennet, 1988). Former secretary of Education, William Bennett, observed there is no evidence that making contraceptive methods more available is the best method for preventing pregnancy. He stated:

> "We currently know very little about how to effectively discourage unmarried teenagers from initiating intercourse ... we do know how to develop character and reinforce good values ... The contraceptive approach is acting with an extravagantly single-minded blindness when it simply, in the name of science, ignores such experience, and offers instead a highly mechanical and bureaucratic solution—more widely available contraceptives in the schools." (p.104)

A public health message from the former Surgeon General C. Everett Koop, stated that the only absolute certain way to prevent AIDS is to be sexually abstinent (Koop, 1988). Koop proposed placing sexuality within the context of marriage and that any health information provided by the federal government should teach children not to engage in sex before they are ready to marry:

"Those of us who are parents, educators, and community leaders, indeed all adults, cannot disregard this responsibility to educate out young. The need is critical and the price of neglect is high. The lives of our young people depend upon our fulfilling our responsibility." (p.130)

Abstinence was brought into the public sphere when, on August 22, 1996, Congress appropriated $50 Million dollars in the Personal Responsibility and Welfare Reform legislation for the promotion of abstinence education for each year from 1998 through 2002. The portion of this funding given to each state was determined by the proportion of the number of low-income children in that state compared to the number of low income children nationally.

In this legislation, the term "abstinence education" was defined as encompassing eight tenets: a) there are social, psychological, and health gains from abstaining from sexual activity; b) abstinence from sexual activity before marriage is the expected standard for all school age children; c) abstinence from sexual activity is the only certain way to prevent out-of-wedlock pregnancy, sexually transmitted disease and other associated health problems; d) a mutually faithful and monogamous relationship in the context of marriage is the expected standard of human sexual activity; e) sexual activity outside of marriage is likely to have harmful psychological and physical effects; f) bearing children out-of-wedlock is likely to have harmful consequences for the child, the parents and society; g) young people need to learn how to reject sexual advances and how alcohol and drug use increases vulnerability to sexual advances; and h) young people need to attain self-sufficiency before engaging in sexual activity (cited in Blinn-Pike, 1999).

When evaluating abstinence-only programs, researchers found among students who had never had sexual intercourse, only 4% of the participants had initiated sexual activity during the follow up session (Howard & McCabe, 1990). A more resent study of abstinence-only programs used with 10,000 students in California demonstrated similar results. Of those students who were virgins before the program, around 13% had initiated intercourse 17 months later (Kirby, Korpi, Barth, & Cagampang, 1997).

Lynn Blinn-Pike (1999) did a study looking at why certain students remained virgins and others did not. For the students who remained abstinent, she found they had absorbed multiple and diverse messages about sex and synthesized them into three distinct factors. The first factor was called *fear-based postponement*. To explain this, one would have to imagine the student saying 'having sex is stupid and I am going to wait because you can get pregnant or die, and besides my parents would kill me.' The second factor is called *emotionality and confusion*. These children would say 'I haven't had sex yet because it might hurt and it is embarrassing and hard to get the stuff you need to protect yourself.' The third factor is for students who have *conservative values*. These students had more traditional values regarding a certain number of life issues. These students who were conservative were also found to live with their parents, they did not drink, had better grades and had better educated fathers. Blinn-Pike (p.300) concludes her study with one simple question. She asks, "What have non-sexually active adolescents done right rather than what have their sexually active peers done wrong?"

Despite the lack of social support of abstinence only programs, enthusiasm for abstinence-only educational programs has increased at the local, state, and federal level (Gahr, 1992). Researchers who found that children who were taught to just "say no to sex" were one-fifth as likely to start having sex as those who did not participate in the program (Griffin, 1993).

While there are several abstinence-only approaches to sex education, there are at least three that have been formerly completed, evaluated and ready for use in the public schools. They are Values and Choices, Teen Aid, and Sex Respect.

• *Values and Choices*: this program includes discussions on self-esteem, self-respect, and the student's own sexuality. It provides "universal" values, which can provide a framework for good decision making. Units on puberty, dating, attraction to the opposite sex, and peer pressure are also offered, along with lessons on the importance of planning for the future, consequences of teenage pregnancy, and understanding sexually transmitted diseases.

- *Teen Aid*: This program includes units on drugs, alcohol, exercise, reproductive anatomy fetal development and childbirth. It also includes lessons on self-esteem, friendship, dating and dealing with peer pressure. Teen Aid advocates the view that a committed and loving marriage is the appropriate context for sexual relationship, along with an understanding of the risks of premarital sexual activity.

- *Sex Respect*: This program focuses on teen sexuality and abstinence and includes the issues of Human Sexuality, sexual freedom and impulsiveness. Units also cover dating, peer pressure, marriage and parenting. Classroom presentations include information on the risks of premarital sex and the benefits of sexual abstinence.

A study was done looking at the attitudes of students who were enrolled in three different sex education programs that emphasized abstinence. The researchers were interested in finding out how the students responded to the programs. Their research found, for the most part, the students responded favorably to the abstinence message. They found that junior-high school student responded more favorably than the high-school students. It is believed the junior-high students had not solidified their opinions and behaviors concerning their own sexuality. They also found the teachers who presented the programs rated it as a positive experience (Olsen, Weed, Nielsen & Jensen, 1992).

"Sex Can Wait"

One program that has been positively evaluated is called *Sex Can Wait*. The *Sex Can Wait* curriculum is said to take a preventative, positive approach with a focus on factors related to early sexual involvement, such as self-esteem, communication, decision making, goal setting and life planning. With this curriculum, the students are actively involved in role-plays, cooperative learning groups, and other learning activities as well as parent-child homework assignment.

The Sex Can Wait curriculum series consists of upper elementary, middle school, and high school components. The program is a five-week abstinence-based sexuality education program consisting of 23 lessons and the upper elementary level and 24 lessons at both the middle and high school levels.

A short term evaluation of the middle school component found a number of positive outcomes, including a decrease in the number of students participating in sexual intercourse in the last 30 days, compared to students in a health class that received their regular curriculum and a "no health" control group (Young, Marx & Core-Gebhart, 1992). A pair of researchers cited this study to say that abstinence programs do not delay the initiation of sexual intercourse. Later, the pair acknowledged this was an inadvertent error on their part and the report actually did find positive changes in recent sexual behavior (Personal communication to Denny, 97).

Later research looked at the effectiveness of the Sex Can Wait curriculum. The results indicated the upper elementary program produced gains in knowledge, more desirable attitudes, and more positive attitudes toward abstinence. At the middle school level, the curriculum produced significant gains in knowledge and more positive attitudes toward abstinence (Denny, Young, Spear, 1999).

In the same research, the middle school level of education was found to have produced an increase in more desirable decision-making behaviors. Several educators have indicated that the development of life skills, such as decision making, should be viewed as an important part of sexuality education program (Denny et al, 1999).

Despite the social atmosphere regarding abstinence-only sex education programs, the results of these studies on Sex Can Wait are encouraging. Educators should consider this curriculum and others interested in educational programs that to help children postpone sexual activity.

I, the author tends to feel that our children are being exposed to too many new stimuli. They are learning too many new things too fast. In the past, there was no Internet, no cell phone, and the children did not have access to various forms on sex information. Today, all kids have to do is just 'log on' and the entire world is open to them at the click of a mouse. This has to change.

Many of the pornographic web sites are free and are accessible to any child any anytime of the night. These companies said there are trying to limit access to these images to requiring the viewer to be over 21. It is tough for the companies to do this because they have no control over who is on the other end of the web connection. The author feels is the parent's responsibility to enforce the rules in the household.

The author also feels it is the parents right to choose how they want their children to be educated around sex. These liberals want comprehensive education where the children learn about gays and lesbians and anal intercourse. What if I don't want that information given to my child. What happens if my child hears that type of information and becomes gay? Who can I blame for that?

Whoever is reading this should see that there are alternatives to the comprehensive education program put forth by liberal organization. As you have just read, many of the children respond favorably to the abstinence message. The parents and the teachers of the program also approve of the program. I do not understand what the problem is. If the children are programmed to wait until marriage for sex, they will be better-adjusted adults who will have very happy lives.

The liberals also want to teach children about safer sex. Since the research has shown that condoms are not 100% effective, I would like to know if Ms. Haffner and her SIECUS colleagues will be available to baby sit my grandchild? I have very strong opinions about this and I do not feel it is appropriate for children to be learning such rubbish. Ms. Haffner likes to quote numbers talking about HIV and teens. Well, the way I see it if the children are not sexually active, they should not have to worry about HIV and pregnancy. One of these days, I would like to sit down with the people at SIECUS and give them all a piece of my mind. That's all I have to say.

9

Dyspareunia

Female dyspareunia has been defined as pain associated with penile-vaginal intercourse. Early clinical descriptions appeared in the Raesseum Papryi IV scrolls of ancient Egypt, which may make dyspareunia one of the earliest recognized sexual dysfunctions (Constatalens & Colorado, 1971). It also may be one of the most common female sexual dysfunction (Fordney, 1978), as well as possibly the most under-reported dysfunction by women (Sarazin & Seymour, 1991), and the sexual dysfunction most commonly linked to physiological pathology (Fordney, 1978).

Until the end of the 19th century, dyspareunia was considered a physical problem of unknown cause which generated very little interest for treatments (Fordney, 1978). With the growth of the psychological sciences in the 20th century, interest in dyspareunia increased only slightly when compared to interest in other sexual dysfunctions. When dyspareunia was examined, the theories on cause usually emphasized the conscious/unconscious motives while ignoring the sensory experience of discomfort. Because of this, dyspareunia was linked to hysteria, which played a major part of women's health care in the first half of the 20th century. While the increase in sexuality research/therapy in the 1960's and 1970's had a major effect in removing dyspareunia from the classification of hysteria, it had very little effect on generating new research and treatment programs (Meana & Binik, 1994).

Classification

Dyspareunia has been described and classified in a number of ways throughout its history as dysfunction. The consistent use of the term 'dyspareunia' started in the 1930's, which was translated from ancient Greek as "difficult mating." (Ellery, 1954).

Dyspareunia is currently defined in the DSM-III-R (1987) as the occurrence of persistent genital pain during or after intercourse. The assessment method used in the study of dyspareunia rarely was more than a simple question: Do you have pain during or after sexual intercourse? Sandberg and Quevillon (1987) claimed that symptoms are universal, with almost every woman at some point experiencing occasional dyspareunia. Fordney (1978) stated that if the pain is only limited to the time of penetration and does not seriously affect desire, receptivity, or orgasm, it should not be considered dyspareunia. Fordney also excluded other possible causes of dyspareunia such as pain from prolonged vaginal intercourse, infections caused my normal bacteria of the vagina or pain caused by the lack of lubrication.

Prevalence

The actual prevalence of dyspareunia is not known. In the 1940's, there were a few studies that looked at prevalence but have now been dismissed due to serious methodological problems. From 1950 to 1969, there were no prevalence studies. The research in the 1970's showed a rather high prevalence in their samples. In clinic studies, it has been claimed that next to anorgasmia, dyspareunia is the most common female sexual dysfunction (Kaplan, 1974; Masters and Johnson, 1970). From the research, the prevalence rate can be anywhere from 4% to 55%.

One of the issues in estimating incidence and prevalence rates for dyspareunia is that many prevalence studies do not include dyspareunia on their list of sexual dysfunctions or do not distinguish it from vaginismus (Bancroft & Coles, 1976). Also, since dyspareunia may exist with another sexual dysfunction, it may not be considered as the main problem (Fink, 1972; Kaplan, 1974).

In spite of the lack of stable research on prevalence, many authors seem to feel the incidence of dyspareunia is increasing (Sarazin & Seymour, 1991; Schellen, 1983). In a literature review of the prevalence of sexual dysfunctions, Spector and Carey (1990) were able to estimate the prevalence to be from 8% to 23%. Most survey research in the 1970's and 1980's appear to confirm the increase but, caution should be taken when interpreting these figures (Meana & Binik, 1994).

In a National sample looking at the prevalence of sexual dysfunctions in the United States, women with dyspareunia made up a smaller group than women with decreased interest in sex, orgasmic problems, lack or pleasure or arousal problems (Laumann, Paik & Rosen, 1999). In a small study by Heim (2001) found that 7% of her sample reported pain during intercourse. In another study of primary care practices by Jamieson and Steege (1996) found that dyspareunia was reported by 46% of sexually active women, with dyspareunia defined as pain during or after intercourse. In another study by Goetsch (1999) found that postpartum dyspareunia was reported by 45% of their sample.

As many as 60% of women experience dyspareunia when the term is broadly defined as episodes of pain with intercourse. Women with symptoms severe enough to require medical attention make up a much smaller group. Many of the women with persistent genital pain do not seek medical attention (Glatt, Zinner & McCormack, 1990).

Causes

The cause of dyspareunia has been divided into two main realms: biological and psychological, with researchers supporting one or the other. Researchers from the psychological camp have claimed the prevalence of psychologically based dyspareunia to be anywhere from low to negligible (Huffman, 1976.) The findings for a psychological cause range from 17% to 70% which shows how unorganized the research actually is (Kresch & Kresch, 1976).

Regarding biological causes, Spano and Lamont (1975) stated that biological causes are usually correctable and seldom the cause of continuing problems. A more resent study looked at chronic pelvic pain and found the same percentage of patients with pain and the control patients with no pain to have biological pathology, with no difference in the type or degree of pathology (Walker, Katon, Harrop-Griffiths, Holm, Russo & Kickoc, 1988). Walker et al.'s research suggests that pathological findings may have little relevance to reported pain.

Patient Characteristics. Consistent traits of people who report dyspareunia are hard to come by. In one study, older age and having a college education were associated with a lower likelihood of dyspareunia. In another study, the incidence of dyspareunia was not associated with age, marital status, race, income or educational level (Jamieson & Steege, 1996).

The most common pain with dyspareunia occurs during coitus, but some women experience pain afterwards, while others report pain at both times (Jamieson & Steege, 1996). The pain reported before intercourse may come from an irritation of the external genitalia or the vasocongestion that occurs during the excitement phase. Women who report dyspareunia were more likely than the general population to report pain with the insertion of a tampon or digit during a gynecological exam (Meana, Binik & Khalife, 1997).

Psychological Issues. Dyspareunia has been correlated with having a more negative attitude towards sexuality, with more sexual function impairment and with lower levels of relationship adjustment (Meana, Binik & Khalife, 1997). Women with dyspareunia were found to have a lower frequency of vaginal intercourse, lower levels of desire and arousal, and to be less orgasmic with oral stimulation and intercourse (Laumann, Paik & Rosen, 1999). Reports of pain with intercourse were associated with low physical and emotional satisfaction, as well as, decreased general happiness. One study found that depression and phobic anxiety were noted more often in patients with dyspareunia compared with control subjects (Meana, Binik & Khalife, 1997). Other studies found no difference from norms with regard to psychopathology, marital adjustment or attitudes towards intercourse (Meana, Binik, Khalife & Cohen, 1997)

Lazarus (1980) provided a breakdown of psychological factors into three categories: developmental, traumatic, and relational.

1. *Developmental factors* refer to early influences on the creation of attitudes towards sexuality. Usually formed in childhood, they set the stage for adult anxiety and fear of the coital experience.

2. *Traumatic factors* refer to a prior aversive coital or sexual experience or some other trauma associated with the genital area.

3. *Relational factors* range from deficits in lovemaking techniques to pervasive feelings that are detrimental to the sexual relationship.

Emotional disturbances going beyond the sexual problem itself was commonly reported for all types of women who report pain during intercourse. Frank (1948) reported that 54.8% of his sample showed "psycho-neuroses", compared with 24.5% of women with biologically caused dyspareunia. To add, Beard et al. (1988) reported that 60% of his sample that complained of dyspareunia and pelvic pain also had emotional disturbances, while Jarvis (1984) felt that depression was a possible cause for dyspareunia. Fordney (1978) claimed that dyspareunic women were no different from any other sexually dysfunctional group. Fordney argued that emotions were clearly in relation to the sexual problem, which appear to be more reactive than causal.

Relationship problems were suggested as a major cause of dyspareunia. One study found that relationship adjustment was inversely related with a dyspareunic pain rating and anxiety and relationship adjustment were significant independent predictors of a dyspareunic pain rating. Depression was not found to be a predictor when patients with dyspareunia were evaluated as a whole (Meana, Binik, Khalife & Cohen, 1998).

Compared to patients with "pelvic pain", patients with dyspareunia did not report a current or previous history of physical or sexual abuse (Laumann, Paik & Rosen, 1999). The role of sexual abuse has been researched but has been dismissed due to methodological flaws.

Biosocial Issues. This idea emphasizes that biological and psychological variables may be interrelated and may work together to maintain symptoms. This idea incorporates social learning and operant conditioning models with pain, psycholgic and physical conditions. For example, using the Operant Conditioning model, the woman does not initially begin with negative expectations, feelings or attitudes. Operant conditioning model supposes that negative events occur (i.e., a woman has a painful sexual experience), which causes a conditioned negative response. This result leads to an increase in dissatisfaction, decreased sexual response and sexual activities become painful. (Meana & Binik, (1994).

Physiological Issues. Even though a high number of biological conditions have been associated with dyspareunia, no study has examined the prevalence of any of these conditions within dyspareunic populations. Dyspareunia is usually viewed as a symptom of a disease instead of an issue in and of itself. It has been stated while looking at the many variables associated with dyspareunia, it is important to keep in mind that dyspareunia is not a symptom of any one disease (Fordney, 1978).

Abarbanel (1978) created categories of possible biological causes as anatomic, pathologic, and iatrogenic. Anatomic causes are congenital or developmental in origin, effecting mainly the introitus and vaginal canal. These would be malformations of the genitals, such as agenesis {failure of a part or organ to develop} of the vagina or the more common case of a rigid hymen. Pathologic causes include acute and chronic infections of the genital tract, pelvic conditions such as endometriosis and malignant/non-malignant growths. Iatrogenic causes are those problems that are caused by a physician, usually as a consequence of an operation such as an episiotomy. Dyspareunia is also common in postmenopausal women who experience vaginal atrophy as a result of hormonal changes (Bachman, Leiblum, Kemmann, Colburn, Schwatzman & Shelden, 1984).

Biological Causes

Entry Dyspareunia. Entry dyspareunia could come from a number of conditions effecting the labia or vestibule. A history of pain with entry is usually associated with vaginismus and inadequate lubrication from the lack of arousal. Entry pain has also been associated with vaginal atrophy, vulvodynia and transient causes such as fungal or bacteria infections. Vaginal atrophy may be caused by inadequate estrogen, which could cause entry pain but, the pain usually, extends into the vaginal canal. On the surface, tenderness along the urethra meatus could suggest urethritis (Steege, Ling, 1993).

In some cases, ulcers and vaginal fissures are visible under inspection. A Herpes infection may cause entry pain. Ulcers that usually go along with Herpes are usually easily identified or the patient may report a history of pervious eruptions with sexual pain limited to times of active infection (Steege, Ling, 1993).

Inadequate Lubrication. The DSM-III-R does not include dyspareunia caused by the lack of lubrication in its definition. This in itself can be problematic in the description of dyspareunia. First, it is hard to determine if a woman is 'lubricating adequately.' Lubrication is not likely to occur in a gynecologist's office. Also, many women may not be able to report their degree of lubrication.

Secondly, there seems to be a high correlation between women low sexual arousal and dyspareunia. Women who are anticipating pain are more likely to be fearful than sexually aroused. Fear interferes with lubrication, which is a major biological part of the sexual arousal pattern. (Meana & Binik, 1994). As was stated earlier, other researchers feel that the most common cause of dyspareunia is the lack of lubrication (Sarazin & Seymour, 1991).

Inadequate lubrication in younger women is usually associated with inhibited arousal phase, but estrogen deficiency seems to be the main cause in older women. Clients who are not getting enough stimulation to the point of arousal should be educated in various foreplay techniques. Problems in the relationship and interpersonal conflict may affect the level of arousal (Anderson & Cyranowski, 1995). What can happen is that the psychological/emotional variables can become a part of a vicious circle. The problem of absent lubrication may first come from unsatisfactory sexual technique, they can become repetitive and an expected part of sex (Halvorsen & Metz, 1992).

Also, surgery for the treatment of chronic pelvic pain can interfere with natural lubrication. If a couple is having trouble with pain due to vaginal dryness, it has been recommended that they try an over the counter water-based lubricant, including Astroglide or Wet (Heim, 2001).

Deep Dyspareunia. The lack of lubrication can lead to problems with dryness and/friction with penile movement. The vaginal barrel may not distend and elongate in response to the arousal phase, and this may cause discomfort, especially in certain positions or with penile impact on the cervix.

The pain that goes with deep thrusting is usually described as 'something being bumped into.' Causes may include endometriosis and pelvic congestion. Ovarian or fallopian tube infections and scarring from pelvic inflammatory disease are less likely to cause pain related to deep dyspareunia. Some women have a retroflexed uterus have also reported deep dyspareunia (Steege & Ling, 1993; DeWitt, 1991).

Postpartum Dyspareunia. The cause for postpartum still remains unclear. One study found that 45% of women had entry pain, a small percentage had pain at the site of the episiotomy repair and 39% reported general genital pain. There was a small difference in pain reported between women who had their first baby and those having their second. Over 25% of these women who had a cesarean section reported having pain, while 41% of lactating women reported dyspareunia. The average time for dyspareunia to stop of the general genital pain group was 5.5 months, and vaginal tenderness lasted up to one year (Goetsch, 1999).

Vaginismus. Vaginismus is caused by a involuntary contraction of the pubococcygeus muscle that surrounds the outer third of the vagina. Vaginismus has been defined many ways and Masters and Johnson defined it as:

> "A psychophysiological syndrome affecting woman's freedom of sexual response by severely, if not totally, impeding sexual function. Anatomically, it involves all components of the pelvic musculature investing the perineum and outer third of the vagina. Physiologically, these muscle groups contract spastically as opposed to their rhythmic contractual response in orgasm experience. This spasm in an involuntary reflex stimulated by imagined, anticipated or real attempts at vaginal penetration." (Masters & Johnson, 1970, p. 113)

It may develop any time psychological or physical pain is related to sexual activity and last for any length of time. Any woman who has experienced sexual trauma can develop vaginismus from psychological causes alone. Vaginismus may have psychological basis, but the problem always has a physical result. This happens because the muscles at the introitus hypertrophy and go into involuntary spasm during sexual activity (Crenshaw & Kessler, 1985).

Theresa Crenshaw from the Crenshaw Clinic in San Diego California defined two types of vaginismus: Primary and Secondary.

Primary Vaginismus—A condition which can be congenital or which develops before a female becomes sexually active. The condition is evident from the first sexual intercourse attempt and often produces unconsummated marriages.

Secondary Vaginismus—A condition acquired as a result of psychological or organic factors occurring after a woman has become sexually active. Pain-free sexual intercourse was an established pattern prior to the development of this condition (Kessler, 1988).

There are a number of pelvic problems that can cause pain with intercourse ranging from constipation resulting in pain with deep thrusting to uterine and cervical infection that result in tenderness in basic pelvic examinations. The act of sexual thrusting in usually more painful than a pelvic examination. Whenever a medical problem develops that causes pelvic pain to last for a length of time, vaginismus will usually develop. It is the body's way to tell the woman "Do not have intercourse anymore, it hurts." The body's self-defense mechanism is to develop a muscular obstruction to intercourse thus making the experience more painful (Crenshaw & Kessler, 1985). In addition to having involuntary muscle spasms of the vaginal orifice, patients with vaginismus are usually fear any sort of vaginal penetration which only adds to their frustration and discomfort (Kaplan, 1974).

Women describe the pain of vaginismus with words such as "ripping," "tearing," "burning," "stinging," or having a "sunburned" vagina. One woman said:

> "I think about sex all the time, not because I have a high sex drive but because it hurts when I have intercourse. As soon as my husband comes home from work, I worry because I'm afraid he'll ask me to make love and I won't want to because of the pain. It isn't that I don't love him. I do. I feel guilty because I am constantly looking for excuses not to have sex with him but I can't help it because it hurts so much. He tried to understand but it's been over a year now and his patience has worn thin. Sometimes he thinks I'm just making it up. I've been to several doctors. When they examine me they say they can't see anything wrong and they tell me to relax. I think they think it's all in my head. Maybe it is, but it still hurts." (Kessler, 1988, p.175)

In some cases, milder feelings, which show the presence of vaginismus, are missed during an examination. For example, if a woman was asked if she had pain during intercourse, she might deny it because the pain is tolerable or "just a discomfort." Because of this, acute forms of vaginismus go undiagnosed and untreated until the condition becomes a problem for the couple's relationship. This could lead to the woman having less intercourse than if there were no discomfort (Crenshaw & Kessler, 1985).

Therapy/Treatment. The standard therapy is a combination of short-term psychotherapy and vaginal dilations. It has been noted that the first and most important step in the treatment of vaginismus is physically showing the existence of the involuntary vaginal spasm to *both* partners (Master & Johnson, 1970).

Vaginal dilations are accomplished by slowly and painlessly inserting lubricated dilators of gradually increasing size into the vagina. The goal is for the woman to be able to painlessly accommodate a dilator that is the equivalent to the girth of the object she and her partner use during intercourse (Kessler, 1988).

Part of the psychological treatment of vaginismus revolves around education. If the woman has learned that sex is supposed to hurt, this will set her up to believe that a woman has to tolerate pain during and discomfort during intercourse. This may cause her to avoid sexual contact, which can create problems in their relationship. It is important for the woman to know that intercourse, including vaginal intromission, is not supposed to hurt (Kessler, 1988).

Interstitial Cystitis. Interstitial Cystitis (IC) is a painful bladder condition characterized by lower abdominal pain, a high frequency and desire to urinate. In its worst state, the desire to urinate can occur as often as every 15 minutes during the day and nearly as often as night (Gillenwater & Wein, 1988).

When the desire to urinate hits a person with IC, the body signals that warn of a full bladder turn into spasms. These spasms may spread causing a dull ache in the lower back. This pain has described as anything from a heaviness to sharp, needle-like, or electrical/shock-like pain. Many women say their pelvic pain is usually located in one specific area. An inflammation and/or pain of the urethra, vulva, or anus has also been reported (Webster & Brennan, 1995). The urine examinations of these women are usually missing harmful bacteria and antibiotic treatments rarely relieve the symptoms (Gillenwater & Wein, 1988). It has been found that 63% of women with IC report dyspareunia as a prominent problem at the onset of IC symptoms (Held, Hanno, Wein, Pauly & Cahn, 1990).

One study reported that patients with IC would have multiple pinpoint hemorrhaged areas within the bladder lining. Depending on the duration and the severity of the symptoms, bladder capacity could range from normal to a small contracted bladder holding only several ounces of fluid. The author of the article recommends a bladder biopsy to rule out bladder cancer (McCormick &Vinson, 1988). Some of the newer areas of research include autoimmunity, deficiency in the bladder lining, and the presence of toxins in the urine (Holm-Bentzen & Lose, 1987).

Sexual problems may be directly related to the symptoms of IC. For example, the need to urinate is a common occurrence during the arousal phase of the sexual response cycle (Caird, 1988). The problem of the high frequency to urinate could lead to the couple becoming sexually frustrated, especially if the woman has to suspend sexual activities to urinate. Also, the fatigue that goes with the lack of sleep and pain is likely to decrease sexual interest. The lack of sexual interest has been reported by 58% of IC patients (Webster & Brennan, 1995).

To add, many IC patients complain of other symptoms. Back pain has been reported by 55% IC patients and joint pain has been reported by 49% of IC patients. However, the biggest issue for IC clients has been reports of dyspareunia (Webster & Brennan, 1995).

Estimates of dyspareunia range from 49% to 65% in IC patients (Held et al., 1990; Webster & Brennan, 1995). A study at Duke University of women with IC-related problems found that 90% of subjects complained of pain related to insertion or deep penetration or post-coital pain. Thirty-five percent reported pain as a response to foreplay and orgasm. Close to 65% said they had pain associated with intercourse either usually or always (Herman, 1989).

It seems that part of the problem in obtaining accurate information lies in the patients' interpretation of the term painful intercourse. One study found that many women indicated that they did not have pain with intercourse because they had stopped having intercourse. Other women wrote they did not have pain during intercourse but reported they had pain the next day and several days afterwards. The author of the study commented this might explain the difference between 48.6% who said they had dyspareunia currently and 68.1% who said intercourse increased their pain (Webster & Brennan, 1995).

There are many reasons why a woman with IC might feel pain during sexual arousal and intercourse. Gillespie (1986) suggested that part of the stress response involves the release of locally irritation neurotransmitters (serotonin, acetlycholine and norpinephrine) into the bladder.

There have also been other explanations for the range of symptoms that are associated with IC. Many women with IC have evidence of inflammation of their urethras, as well as, their bladders. This group of women may have pain during or after urination, where other IC patients will feel relief after urinating. It seems like any type of pressure on the abdomen would increase the pain of women who has pelvic pain where manipulation or pressure near the urethra may cause pain for those who have a urethral disease (McCormick & Vinson, 1988).

Any source of vasocongestion, including sexual arousal, might increase feelings to urinate, as well as, pain in some women. Orgasm seems to relieve the congestion for some but in others, orgasm may be painful in itself or result in post-coital pain. Over time, due to negative sexual experiences, these women may develop an anxiety about sexual activities, which could lead to inadequate lubrication. Intercourse without adequate lubrication has been found to increase the possibility of "trauma" during intercourse (Webster, 1993).

Other medical problems could contribute to the sexual problems for women with IC. These include vulvodynia and vestibulitis. It seems the causes of these problems are hard to find, but several researchers have noted that patients with IC may also suffer from these inflammatory conditions of the vulva and vaginal vestibule (Fitzpatrick & DeLancey, Elkins, & McGuire, 1993). With postmenopausal women, estrogen may result in a friable {brittle} vaginal canal and urethral tissue, and decreased vaginal lubrication. Also, medication used to treat IC such as antihistamines, antidepressants, and central nervous system depressants, may provide another source for decreased sexual interest and/or difficulty experiencing orgasm (McCormick, 1995; Webster, 1993).

Therapy/Treatment. One of the most commonly used strategies includes urinating before and after intercourse. Others include avoiding intercourse when having symptoms, avoiding pressure on the urethra, trying sexual positions besides the missionary position and not having intercourse if there is insufficient lubrication. Many couples use Astroglide to aid with natural lubrication (Webster & Brennan, 1995). Pre-menopausal women reported not using diaphragms, probably because of the pressure placed on the bladder (Webster, 1996).

Other researchers found that avoiding spicy foods, caffeine, and carbonated drinks can reduce their symptoms. It has also been recommended that these women avoid cheeses, chocolate, bananas, and red wine (Gillespie, 1986).

Warm baths or hot pads on the pubis and back may add increase comfort in patients. Wearing loose clothing can also reduce pressure on the bladder. Vigorous exercise should be avoided because it can be irritating to the bladder. Also, ways of reducing arousal associated with the pain can be helpful for IC patients. Methods that have been reported as effective include meditation, prayer, progressive relaxation, visualization, and self-hypnosis (Chaiken, Blaivas & Blaivas, 1993).

Vulvodynia/Vestibilitis. Vulvodynia is a syndrome of unexplained genital pain that is usually accompanied by physical disabilities, sexual dysfunction and limitations of daily activities. The age distribution for the condition may range from 20s to the 60s, and seems to be limited almost exclusively to white women (Friedrick, 1987).

Of women who report Vulvodynia, sexual risk taking is usually unremarkable and few patients have a history of sexually transmitted infection (Paavonen, 1995). The genital pain usually has an acute onset. In many cases, the genital pain becomes chronic lasting for months to years. This pain is usually described as a burning or sting-ing, or feeling of rawness or irritation (McKay, 1989).

Many patients visit several doctors before being diagnosed. Many of these women are treated with topical medications, which usually offers very little help. In some cases, inappropriate medications may make the symptoms worse (McKay, 1991). Vaginal cultures are usu-ally negative. With few outward physical symptoms, patients are usu-ally told the problem is mental therefore dismissing their pain and adding to their overall distress (Gottleb, 1995).

The chronic pain itself may cause psychological distress to a woman and her partner (Turner & Marinoff, 1991). The couples' relationship may be threatened when the pain is misunderstood as an alibi for avoiding sexual activities. Anxiety and depression, which could may be increased by long-term pain, could lead to a diagnosis of "psychogenic pain". Even worse, because of this label, the woman could be considered to be the cause and not the victim of her situa-tion (Butcher, 1999).

Subsets of Vulvodynia. Recently, there have been several subsets of vulvodynia identified. It has been stated that certain subsets may also co-exist with others. For proper treatment, a doctor should accurately identify them.

- Vulvar Vestibulitis. This syndrome is characterized by entry dys-pareunia, discomfort at the opening of the vagina, vaginal tender-ness and having a 'redness' at the vaginal opening (McKay, 1991).

- Cyclic Vulvovaginitis. This is believed to be the most common cause of vulvodynia. It is believed to be caused by a hypersensitivity to Candida. The pain is typically worse just before or during men-strual bleeding. The pain may be even worse after intercourse, especially the following day (Ashman & Ott, 1989).

- Dysesthetic Vulvodynia. This type usually appears in women who are peri—or postmenopausal. The pain that occurs in this subtype is a constant burning pain that is not cyclic (McKay, 1993).

- Vulvar Dermatoses. This subtype causes itching and in some cases pain, which may be accompanied by scaly lesions. Erosions or ulcers may come from excessive scratching. (McKay, 1991).

Therapy/Treatment. Cyclic cases are thought to be caused by yeast infection, which can be detected at times and not detected in others. Treatment of the cyclic cases may include an anti-candidal medication even if vaginal cultures are negative. Severe or stubborn cases may be treated with laser therapy (McKay, 1989).

Laser surgery should be used in cases were all other forms of treatment have failed. Surgery should be used in patients whose pain has lasted for more that six months, prevents sexual intercourse and patients who have undergone a specific treatment for a subset of vulvodynia where no cause can be found (Marinoff & Turner, 1991). Surgical removal of vulvar tissue has been reported to alleviate symptoms in up to two-thirds of patients (Mann, Kaufman, Brown & Adam, 1992).

What Do I Think?

For the longest time, I was struggling to pick a topic. I remember sitting in the library picking my brain for an interesting topic. I came up with a few but the desire faded fast. Then I said to if I can spell dyspareunia correctly, I would stay with it as a topic. I did a search and it came back with several articles {so I must have spelled it correctly}. Now, I am glad I did because there are a few things that disturb me.

As I was doing the literature search and writing this paper, I was thinking about how confusing this could be for a woman who goes into to see a doctor because of genital pain. I have the feeling that most general practitioners have no clue what dyspareunia is. If they have heard of it, I believe it is not likely they are familiar with all of the possible causes. In this paper, I only really focused on the biological problems and barely even touched the psychological. What I am really afraid of is how an uninformed doctor would just dismiss her complaints as being mental. To add, due to physician's lack on education regarding sexual matters, this can only increase the likelihood of dyspareunia being misdiagnosed as mental problem. Unless the doctor can *see* something that has the potential to cause pain, I just have this feeling they would choose the easy answer. In a situation like this, I guess the best case scenario would be if the woman were referred to a specialist/ob-gyn who had experience in dealing with these matters.

I was reading another book for Bill Stayton's class when I came across to example of how uninformed physicians can do harm. This example revolves around Robin, a woman who was seeking treatment for vaginismus. Robin's female doctor said she did not "see any blockage or anything wrong with you but your opening is very, very small. (Leiblum & Rosen, p.190). Then, she went to a new gynecologist who also had problems with the genital examination on Robin. He asked her if she had sexual intercourse and she said no. He said he could not do the examination because her "... opening is too small. You may have a problem because your opening is too small. Try to get aroused first." (Leiblum & Rosen, p.191). The doctor did not offer her any other assistance or referrals. This is what I was afraid of.

As I was writing this paper, I was really thinking about how many possible cases of dyspareunia there could be among Black women in America. For the past few years, I have been stuck on the effect of stereotypes in the Black community and this has the potential to be huge.

For example, one of the biggest stereotypes is that all Black men have a large penis. Now, relate that to vaginal intercourse. Lets say the woman in not producing an adequate amount of lubrication due to low estrogen levels. During the act, she begins to feel pain but equates that to his penis size. I think she may suffer through the pain and never realize its actually has a biological cause.

Another example could be pain located around her cervical area (deep dyspareunia). I believe the woman would be more inclined to tolerate that pain/discomfort than to complain do to the stereotype. When I used to give health presentations, I can clearly remember women telling me about their discomfort when their partner's penis would bump into their cervix. I used to tell them to go to the doctor just to make sure everything was ok but, they would dismiss the pain and say their partner had a large penis.

For women in general regardless of race, I see thousands on women 'suffering in silence'. I blame this on society's view of sexuality. To me, the message is women's sexuality should be kept silence. There is the old saying that girls are taught about their elbows, arms, and bellybuttons but are rarely ever told where their clitoris is. Do you see my point?

Now, there is Viagra. The point of sexuality in this country seems to be focused on creating the male erection and helping it to stay up at all costs. I would bet there is a correlation between the appearance of Viagra and an increase in reports of dyspareunia among women. I would have to say that there needs to be a vocal spokesperson who has the ability to raise national awareness regarding dyspareunia in women. Bob Dole is the poster boy for erectile dysfunction. There should be a woman/women who has national visibility like him. Has anyone ever talked to Elizabeth Dole regarding genital pain during sex?

10

Rapid Ejaculation

For many couples, the male's ability to control the timing of his ejaculation is a major part of his and his partner's sexual pleasure. If ejaculation happens before it is desired, it can be disappointing and could lead to other sexual problems including erectile difficulties, female anorgasmia, low sexual desire, and sexual aversion (Rust et al., 1988).

Over 30 years ago, Masters and Johnson (1970) said "premature ejaculation [could] be brought fully under control in our culture during the next decade" (p.359). But, ejaculating sooner than desired remains the most common male issue, effecting as many as one-third to three-quarters (Spector & Carey, 1990) of men, regardless of their orientation.

Kinsey (et. al, 1948) rejected the idea the most men would want to learn to delay ejaculation. Kinsey and his group considered rapid ejaculation an adaptive response, rather than a sexual dysfunction:

> "It would be difficult to find another situation in which an individual who was quick and intense in his responses was labeled anything but superior, and that in most instances is exactly what they rapidly ejaculating male is" (p.580).

In Western cultures, as many as 60% of men wish to prolong latency to orgasm (Reading & Wiest, 1984) and rapid ejaculation causes many men and their partners psychological distress. To add, rapid ejaculation is still one of the most common complaints from men and couples seeking therapy (Kaplan, 1974).

Definitions

There seems to be a lack of consistency regarding the definition of rapid ejaculation. Within the field, there is confusion and an overall disagreement over what exactly constitutes rapid ejaculation. Some of the definitions have been based quantitative dimensions of intercourse such as the number of thrusts, length of intercourse, partner satisfaction and voluntary control. To add, many of these definitions are sexist, heterosexist, and coitally focused (Grenier & Byers, 1995).

The DSM-IV (Diagnostic and Statistical Manual of Mental disorders, American Psychiatric Association [APA], 1994, p. 509) has its own definition of the sexual disorder. The DSM-IV defines rapid ejaculation by three criteria. They involve:

1. A persistent or recurrent ejaculation with minimal sexual stimulation before, upon, or shortly after penetration and before the person wishes.

2. The disturbance must cause marked distress or interpersonal difficulty.

3. The premature ejaculation is not due exclusively to the direct effects of a substance.

The DSM-IV includes three subtype specificers: lifelong versus acquired, generalized versus situational, and psychological versus combined etiology. One of the problems is the fact that the DSM-IV does not define any component of the description (Rowland et al, 2001).

Quantitative Methods

One method defined rapid ejaculation in terms of the number of intra-vaginal thrusts before ejaculation (Colpi et al., 1986). This method does have the advantage of being quantifiable and objective. One group defined rapid ejaculation as ejaculation before 15 vaginal thrusts. Others used 8 vaginal thrusts as their definition. One of the problems with their definitions was that neither group offered any reason for their number of thrusts. Also, they did not define what a "thrust" consisted of along variables, which include speed, vigor or depth (Grenier & Byers, 1995).

Another idea to define rapid ejaculation revolved around the time between intromission and ejaculation. Rapid ejaculation has been defined as ejaculating within 1 minute (Cooper & Magnus, 1984), 2 minutes (Spiess at al., 1984), 3 minutes (Strassberg et al., 1987), 4 minutes (LoPiccolo, 1978), 5 minutes (Kilmann and Auerbach, 1979), and 7 minutes (Schover at al., 1982). It was rare for any rationale to be given but LoPiccolo (1978) felt that ejaculation before 4 minutes after intromission was rapid based on Gebhard's (1966) finding that the average duration of intercourse lasted between 4 and 7 minutes.

What is interesting was the average length of intercourse might not represent the desired length of satisfactory intercourse. Darling (et al., 1991) found in their survey of women that the preferred length of intercourse was over 11 minutes.

One main problem was that those definitions based on the number of thrusts may increased sexual anxiety and spectatoring, and may even promote goal-oriented sexual behavior. To add, using a cutoff score tends to distort groups because men who are similar would be assigned to different groups. For example, in using 2 minutes as a cut off time, people could be placed into different groups. If one man ejaculated in 1:30 seconds, he would be defined as have rapid ejaculation but, a man who ejaculated in 2:15 would not (Grenier & Byers, 1995).

Voluntary Control

Some researchers and therapists started to define rapid ejaculation in terms of voluntary control (Kaplan, 1974). If a man was unable to voluntarily delay his ejaculation, he was diagnosed as having a rapid ejaculation. Defining rapid ejaculation in these terms eliminated the need for a performance standard like time or the number of thrusts.

One problem has been the fact that the definition has not been defined well enough that allow it to be compared to other subjects or research. A second problem with the definition is the lack of clarity about what men are supposed to have voluntary control over. Kaplan (1974) felt that men who have control have control over the actual reflex that causes ejaculation. To add, Levine (1992) felt that men with poor control failed to raise their "threshold for the reflex sequence of orgasm" (p.91). There seems to be a lack a research that shows that the ejaculatory reflex can be brought under voluntary control. Nor has it been demonstrated that men who have control are actually controlling their ejaculatory reflex (Grenier & Byers, 1995).

Latency and Control

Grenier and Byers (1993) looked at the sexual and ejaculatory behavior in university men. They found that ejaculatory latency and perceived ejaculatory control were weakly related. They found that men with long ejaculatory latencies and men with short latencies did not report having poor ejaculatory control.

Strassberg (et al, 1990) defined a man as having a rapid ejaculation if, during at least 50% of his attempts at intercourse, he:

1.   Felt he had little voluntary control over when he ejaculated, and

2.   He ejaculated within 2 minutes or less after intromission.

This definition was thought to be an improvement over some of the earlier definitions because it says that rapid ejaculation may have separate variables such as control and latency. But at the same time, this definition falls back into using cutoff points and the idea of voluntary control (Grenier & Byers, 1995).

Causes

Early Experiences

Masters and Johnson (1970) suggested that early conditioning could be a cause of rapid ejaculation. The idea was those men whose early experiences that were characterized by haste and nervousness were conditioned to ejaculate rapidly. They felt that it only took two or three "events" of rushed intercourse before a pattern of rapid ejaculation appeared.

Williams (1984) described four cases of men who had ejaculatory control but developed secondary rapid ejaculation. Williams believed these men had taught themselves to ejaculate quickly due to their perception their partner was not sexually interested. Later, when these men wanted to prolong intercourse they were unable because of the learned behavior.

Psychodynamic Explanation

There have been two psychodynamic explanations for the cause of rapid ejaculation. Ellis (1936) felt that the main cause of rapid ejaculation was excessive narcissism during infancy that resulted in an exaggerated importance being placed on the penis and the associated with the pleasure of urination.

Kaplan (1974) felt the rapid ejaculation was caused by an unconscious, deep-seated hatred of women. The idea was by ejaculating quickly, the man 'soils' the women and also robs her of sexual pleasure. In 1989, Kaplan said most of the men do not have personality disorders, thus reversing her earlier psychodynamic explanation.

Anxiety

One theory is that rapid ejaculation was caused by a high level of anxiety (Zilbergeld, 1987). There are two basic ideas about how anxiety causes rapid ejaculation. The first idea is that increased anxiety activates the sympathetic nervous system, the same system that is responsible for the emission of ejaculate (Wolpe, 1982). A study by Kockott (et al., 1980) found that high anxiety men showed more sex avoidance behavior and only ejaculated rapidly during intercourse. The low anxiety men ejaculated rapidly during both intercourse and masturbation and showed less sex avoidance.

The second idea suggests that men with high levels of anxiety are distracted during sexual activity by thought about performance and sexual adequacy. It is the distracting thoughts that prevent the man from monitoring his level of arousal or feeling the beginning sensations of ejaculation. So, what is thought to happen is that the ejaculation essentially "sneaks up" on the man so that he is unable to control the timing of his ejaculation (Kaplan, 1974; Zilbergeld, 1987).

Amount of Sexual Activity

Some researchers felt that men who experience rapid ejaculation have lower frequencies of sexual activity than men without rapid ejaculation (Gospodinoff, 1989). It could be that increased sexual activity leads to an increased awareness of sensations leading up to ejaculation, an increased ejaculatory threshold and decreased penile sensitivity. It could be that men who know they ejaculate rapidly avoid sex because of their embarrassment or anxiety about their lack of control. There are some studies that show rapid ejaculation is related with less frequent sexual activity (Gospodinoff, 1989) but, other studies that do not find that relationship (Strassberg et al., 1987).

Technique

Zilbergeld (1978) felt that ejaculatory control was a result of conscious or unconscious techniques that were effective in delaying ejaculation. He asked men with good ejaculatory control how they delayed ejaculation. After these men monitored their sexual behavior and they said they did make changes in their behavior so they could delay ejaculation. The men said these changes included "squeezing or relaxing the pelvic muscles, slowing the tempo, changing the depth of thrusting or changing the type of thrusting" (p.262).

Penile Sensitivity

There are theories that men with rapid ejaculation ejaculate quickly because their penises have a greater sensitivity to stimulation and therefore, reach the critical level of stimulation required to ejaculate (Strassberg et al, 1990). It has been found that young men have greater penile sensitivity than older men (Rowland et al., 1989) which has been used to explain the incidence of primary rapid ejaculation in younger men. But at the same time, the increased incidence in younger men could be a result of greater anxiety, less frequent sexual activity and fewer chances to learn ejaculatory control (Gospodinoff, 1989).

Ejaculatory Reflex

Some authors felt that a malfunctioning ejaculatory reflex causes rapid ejaculation. The squeeze technique developed by Semans (1965), which could be the most widely used treatment method for rapid ejaculation, is based on the idea of a malfunctioning ejaculatory reflex. Other researchers felt that men with rapid ejaculation have a hypersensitivity that makes them ejaculate faster (Colpi et al., 1986). Gospodinoff (1989) hypothesized that a faster bulbocavernosus reflex (BCR; i.e., the expulsion reflex) may interfere with the learning process men undergo when learning to control their ejaculation. It is the bulbocavernosus muscle surrounds the urethral bulb and is one of the muscles responsible for the expulsive phase.

Treatments

The Stop/Start Technique

In 1956, Semans came up with the basic procedure of the stop/start technique. When using this to control rapid ejaculation, the man in repeatedly brought to high levels of arousal and them stimulation is stopped just before ejaculation begins. Then in 1970, Masters and Johnson came up with a slight variation on the stop/start technique called the Squeeze technique. The difference is when his orgasm is approaching and stimulation is stopped, the man or his partner squeezes the penis just below the frenulum with the thumb and fore-finger. The loss of stimulation along with the squeezing of the penis stops the process of ejaculation and could lead to a partial or total loss of erection.

In 1978, LoPiccolo modified the stop/start technique. The idea was that in addition to stopping stimulation, the man should also pull down on his scrotum when nearing ejaculation. The idea was this would reverse the physiological process of the elevation of the testicles, which normally happens before ejaculation and should stop ejaculation.

Another variation put forth by LoPiccolo was the Valsalva Maneuver. This behavior was described as the man to force an exhalation when the airway is closed. The rationale for this intervention is that this could induce stimulation in the sympathetic nervous system which should counteract the process of ejaculation (LoPiccolo, 1978).

Zilbergeld (1978) added that the stop/start techniques provided men with rapid ejaculation to explore changes in sexual behavior that they had not considered previously or perhaps needed permission to change. He felt the technique might change their sexual behavior enough to allow men with rapid ejaculation to find new ejaculatory delaying methods that were already known to men with good ejaculatory control.

Masters and Johnson (1970) reported a failure rate of 2.2% within a sample of 186 men. More recent studies found a much lower success rate using the stop/start technique. Kilmann (et al., 1986) found an average success rate of 62% for treatment of rapid ejaculation. Hawton and Catalan (1986) reported that only 64% of clients gained ejaculatory control after using the squeeze technique. In addition, they found that only one-third of those men showed continued control at 3 years post-treatment. DeAmicis (et al., 1985) found that all of the post-therapy gains were lost at a 3-year follow-up.

Drugs

There a few classes of drugs that have been useful in delaying ejaculation. Some drugs interfere with the sympathetic nervous systems' activation of the ejaculatory reflex and other drugs that increase the level of serotonin.

Alpha-adrenergic blockers that are used in the treatment of rapid ejaculation are believed to work because it is the sympathetic nervous system that is responsible for the movement of seminal fluids through the genital duct system. This would prevent the accumulation of fluid near the posterior urethra thus delaying the activation of the nervous system which causes the expulsive phase of ejaculation (Shilon et al, 1984). Shilon's own research found that 50% of the men reported increased ejaculatory latencies. It was also reported that some of the side effects of alpha-blocker included having 'dry ejaculations'.

Segraves (1989) believed that serotonin played a role in stopping the neurotransmission required for the ejaculatory reflex to work. Assalian (1991) reported clomipramine, a drug that increases levels of serotonin, resulted in ejaculatory latencies in 100% of the subjects with rapid ejaculation. Segraves (et al, 1992) reported ejaculatory latencies in 70%of men with rapid ejaculation using clomipramine. Colpi (et al., 1986) mentioned they had also successfully treated primary rapid ejaculation with clomipramine. It should be noted that clomipramine has been associated with painful intercourse (Aizenberg et al, 1991), anorgasmia (Montiero et al., 1987), and erectile dysfunction (Beaumont, 1973).

In another study, men were given paroxetene (Paxil). In the men who took paroxetene, their ejaculatory latency increased 7-10 minutes and they also described an increased libido. These same men also reported increased sexual satisfaction and an increase in partner satisfaction (Althof, 1995). Ruff and St. Lawrence (1985) reported that some doctors were using topical anesthetics applied to the penis penile sensation and thereby increasing ejaculatory latencies.

Premature Ejaculation: Nature's Plan

One of the more interesting theories I came across had to do with speedy ejaculation as a passed on genetic trait. It was hypothesized that quick ejaculation was advantageous in the past. It is believed that the trait of premature ejaculation was passed on to more and more generations because it was an evolutionarily successful strategy. It seems that premature ejaculation has become a dysfunction only in recent times (Hong, 1984).

With some exceptions such as dogs and foxes, sexual intercourse within mammals is usually over quickly. The duration of sexual intercourse is measured in minutes and in many cases in seconds (Diakow, 1974). In has been found that human males, with average speed of 2 minutes, are relatively slow when compared with other species. Men are only second to the orangutan among all the great apes in ejaculatory control (Hong, 1984).

To begin to explain this theory, there seems to be a relation between the speed of intercourse and male aggression. This idea states where the time between intromission and ejaculation is long, there is a tendency for male violence.

There was a time when male proto-humans had variations in their speed of copulation. Some of these males could mount and ejaculate fairly quickly. It was thought that these males were less bothersome to their female partners and not viewed as competition by other males. Because of their ability to copulate quickly, this gave them the chance to have sex with a greater number of females. Therefore, the rapid ejaculators had more sex and more chances to impregnate which lead to an increased chance of their 'rapid genes' to be passed onto the next generation.

After a literature review, Lancaster (1979) concluded among non-human primates, the single most important factor of high status was maturity, not fighting ability or social aggressiveness. Those young proto-humans that were fast may have a better chance of reaching maturity in better health. Therefore, they would be in a better position to reach alpha status. These 'rapid males' would have more sexual access and reproduce more of their own kind. Lancaster concluded that the ancestry of Homo sapiens became overpopulated with rapid ejaculators.

Hong supported Lancaster by stating because of their rapid ejaculation, there was less chance for being injured by other males. This also meant they might live longer giving them more opportunities to have offspring that would carry their 'rapid genes'. It is believed as this trait was passed along from generation to generation therefore, natural selection produced more and more males who ejaculated quickly (Hong, 1984).

The question was if rapid ejaculation was advantageous in the past, why is it labeled as a dysfunction today? Even the term premature ejaculation has a negative connotation because it indicates bad timing. It seems that the duration of intercourse did not become a major clinical issue until the past 2 decades or so. Ehrentheil (1974) attempted to find literature on premature ejaculation before the 20th century but was unsuccessful.

The primary function of sex was for procreation and the secondary function was for recreation (Foote, 1954). As long as sex was considered as a means for reproduction, the idea of female pleasure was left out of the equation. It seems this became a problem around the 1960s. The availability of contraceptives and women's awakened awareness regarding their sexuality decrease the importance of procreation. Therefore, coming from a Freudian mindset, a male's speed of reaching an orgasm has become an issue. The whole issue could be the result of biology failing to keep up with social change or social change taking humans away from their natural biology (Hong, 1984).

My Thoughts

Since I am a want-to-be therapist, I felt it would be a good idea to look at the number one complaint of men. I am sure as I go along my career in therapy, I am sure I will come across this more than once. But, I do have some problems with a few of things I read and wrote about.

First off, the definitions seem to be all over the place. Some people use time, others use the number of thrusts, etc. It is a bit crazy. Of course, I came up with my own definition. I think that limiting rapid ejaculation to just one variable creates it own problems. I really believe that the definitions caused more problems than they helped to fix. What happens if rapid ejaculation occurs every so often? For example, let's say a man, using his own definition, rapidly ejaculated 3 out of every ten times. Is he rapid?

I say the definition should be made up of a number of variables. For example, I feel the definition should include:

1. the persons own definition, and

2. Whether it is affecting his relationship, and

3. The sexual satisfaction of the partner.

Secondly, I feel the causes I found were pretty interesting. Out of them all, I seem to agree with early experiences linked with anxiety. For example, if the young male {teenager} was having sex at home, there was chance of being caught. That had to increase the overall levels of anxiety. Also, I think quick ejaculatory experience with masturbation could also play a role. From my understanding, many men rush to ejaculate which I feel could teach them to ejaculate quickly when with a partner as well. I feel if men were taught a new technique where they could feel their ejaculation starting {stop/start}, they could move that technique over to partnered sexual activity.

Third, I am not a big fan of taking drugs for treatment. As you read, some of them have bad side effects, which may do more harm than good. I like the stop/start technique minus the testicle pulling. Yes, I understand the bio-mechanics of the testicles rising before ejaculation but that just sounds painful and I think could lead to erection problems. Using a combination of sensate focus linked with the start/stop technique should be helpful. The part that concerns me is that the couple would have to make time to work on it. If they don't do the work, the problem may continue indefinitely and possibly harm the relationship.

Forth, the last piece I cited about rapid ejaculation as nature's plan was interesting. I think the author made a good case but times have changed. Maybe in the past, being a rapid ejaculator may have had its advantages but again, times have changed. So, let's say I am genetically predispositioned to be a rapid ejaculator. Eliminating genetic resequencing, is there really anything I could do about it? It's not like I can practice changing my eye color or my height. It is an interesting idea but.... nah, it just does not work for me.

11

Female Circumcision:
Alive and Well in the
United States
(Hypothetically)

The topic of this article deals with patriarchal social scripts and the negative influence they have over the women in this society. In various parts of the world, women are subjected to methods of sexual control including female circumcision (genital mutilation is a more correct term). In this country, women are subjected to a variation of circumcision I call "social circumcision." In this article, I hope to explain how this patriarchal culture socializes women to fear and dislike their own bodies and come to depend on males for their sexual well being.

Background

To understand the present, it is necessary to understand what female circumcision is and why it is practiced. Female circumcision is practiced in some parts of Africa, Asia and Australia. The procedure varies between the removal of the clitoral hood to the removal of the clitoris and the labia minora entirely and also parts of the labia majora. The most severe form of this practice is called infibulation or 'pharaonic' circumcision where all of the external genitalia are removed (Slack, 1988). In these cultures, the vagina is then held closed with thorns or stitches. The woman's vagina is supposed to remain "sealed" until she becomes a bride when the husband uses his penis or a knife to "reopen" her. (Shaw, 1985) A woman may be re-sealed and re-opened numerous times according to the will of her husband.

Medical problems run rampant because of the operation. Shock is very common because anesthesia is rarely used. Damage to other organs is also a problem. In some circumstances, animal dung is used to stop the bleeding so infections are also a problem. If the vagina is sealed incorrectly, menstrual fluid and urine cannon be released (Dysmenorrhea). Therefore, the woman may have to have the operation a second time. For women who have been infibulated, child birth can be a life threatening experience. Since the hardened scar tissue does not stretch, vaginal tearing or a ruptured uterus are common. (Slack, 1988)

One should ask with the pain and obvious danger involved, why is this practiced? There are several reasons. These reasons are based strictly on patriarchal beliefs that have affected large areas of the world. Males of this culture have long had an obsession with the female genitals. First, female circumcision is supposed to ensure the woman is "pure" when she becomes a bride. (Giorgis, 1981) This form of double talk, the use of the word "pure", is given an enlightened flavor as is to say being clean is akin to being a goddess, so the operation will make them a better human being. Interestingly enough, it is contact with a male that can make her unclean. It makes the predatory male not responsible for this uncontrollable action. Because men define appropriate controls, it would be unthinkable to stitch the penis to the stomach with a flexible thorny branch where the male is punished for getting an erection. That tactic would control the 'uncontrollable' actions and keep women "pure" (males as well!) however, the goal is to control women's sexual behavior, the not the behavior of men.

Secondly, certain religious customs call for the removal of the clitoris. In these cultures, the clitoris is seen as being ugly and is said to interfere with intercourse (Giorgis, 1981). The only reason this clitoris is seen as being ugly is because male do not and will never have one. If male were born with a clitoris, it would be viewed as the most beautiful organ on the planet (just like the penis already is). The same way men use their penile length to estimate everything from intelligence to social power, they measure the sensitivity of their clitoris as being a fully functioning male: He whose clitoris is the most sensitive wins!

Third, the removal of the clitoris is said to reduce a woman's sexual desire (Giorgis, 1981). It would seem that the all-powerful male is afraid of the woman's sexual capacity. So, the male call for the removal of the part of the body that is extremely important in female sexuality and sexual pleasuring. The males found out that female have a higher sexual capacity than they did. That was seen as a direct threat to their patriarchal penile power. So, the 'penilly' (mortally) wounded male decided to reclaim his almighty status by punishing woman for out performing them sexually. These beliefs have been around for hundreds of years and are being cast upon women today.

In explaining female circumcisions longevity, Barbara Reynolds (Reynolds, 1994) felt it has to do with male status. "It's patriarchal", she says, "relating to slavery, and designed to maintain polygamy for men and monogamy for women." Male realized "real men" are not supposed to let things get out of control and maintain the protective ideology of social control. Men are afraid of an egalitarian society because they give up their control. Therefore, males must control everything and if the slightest hole in patriarchy (e.g., women's sexual liberation), female circumcision was created to maintain patriarchy. That is why men are forced into a protective position. Mary Daly (1978) states the clitoris is seen as "… impure because it does not serve male purpose. It has not necessary function in reproduction." (p.159). Since it serves not usefulness except for female pleasure, it is a useless organ. If males had as organ that was stimulated by the clitoris, males would have created a drug or a "special surgery" to increase the size of the clitoris. Notice the male still does not have to ingest any drugs or submit to any operations.

Male Defined Sexuality

In patriarchal cultures, males get to decide what is sexual and whose responsibility it is to "turn on" the other sexually. In the United States, women are supposed to be large busted with small waists with even smaller minds to be considered "sexy." Women follow these rules by dieting themselves into non-existence and mutilating their bodies with plastic surgery trying (being forced) to become the ultimate male fantasy. To add, in this country, we have our own form of foot binding by saying to women—who wears the highest heeled shoes will be the "societal Cinderella."

By socializing women to believe the way they appear naturally is not good enough, the women loose themselves by trying to conform. The male buys the push-up bras and etcetera to create the image he wishes she was. She was given the job of turning him on sexually. I would dare to call this the Third Shift.

Social Circumcisions

On this patriarchal planet, women are a taught to view their sexuality as something negative. In Africa and other physically circumcising countries, the women's clitoris and sometimes other parts of the female genitals are removed. This is done to perpetuate the patriarchal ideology. Here, in America, women suffer emotional, not physical circumcision. Women are socialized to regard their sexuality and genitals in a negative light. I propose the term "Social Circumcision"—the socialization of women to disregard their sexuality in order to be accepted by the dominant culture. Women, who have been 'circumcised' in this fashion, therefore, delegate their sexual pleasure to the male. Males have been socialized to follow certain sexual scripts that usually do not involve too much in the area of female pleasure. Since the clitoris is viewed as an unnecessary organ, the male bypasses her pleasure in exchange for his own and she allows his pleasure at the expense of her own.

First, men are socialized that women's sexual pleasure is unimportant. Secondly, women themselves are socialized to view their sexuality as something negative. This is the basis for the patriarchal sexuality defense—teach males incorrectly about sex and teach females nothing about their sexuality. Since women are cut off from their sexuality, patriarchy maintains its control and inhibits women from becoming: Themselves.

The Unimportant Clitoris

The notion that the clitoris is unimportant is buried deep within this culture. As children, females are taught to point to their nose, mouth and tummy but, it would be unheard of that they would be taught where their clitoris is. That is how patriarchy first takes hold over the person. At early ages, you are already taught that someone else will educate you with your sexual boundaries. It only makes sense that this information comes from the parents who have become thoughtless automatons following the unspoken words of the patriarchy (society). They, the parents, do not know any better. It is not until later in life that the female will stumble across her clitoris.

It is interesting to mention that masturbation in females usually begins with an "accidental discovery" (Clifford, 1978)—the discovery of the clitoris. This shows one important fact. Social Circumcision, just like socialization, takes place over a period of time. Even though women have been socialized not to explore their bodies, most women are questioning their early training. Social Circumcision is an extremely powerful force though. Even after the woman has discovered her clitoris, it is likely she will socialize her own daughter(s) to follow the patriarchal rule. When the next generation is socialized, this pre-programmed automates pseudo-self emerges.

Moving forward to adult partnered sexual activity, research shows that clitoral stimulation is more important that vaginal stimulation in achieving orgasm (Master, Johnson, 1966). Women who have engaged in two person sexual activities probably realize this fact. But, since the clitoris is viewed as an unnecessary organ in regard to male pleasure, that could explain why the male focuses on penile-vaginal interaction. Patriarchal sexual scripts have socialized both males and females to believe that 'real women' orgasm fro penile thrusting and nothing more. This is a belief that originated from the mind of Freud and was also adopted into the patriarchal sexual script. It is basically saying it is a woman's fault if she cannot orgasm from thrusting. Again, males are placing the blame on women and having orgasm via the clitoris is looked down upon.

Research shows that men desire coitus more frequently while women desire more "foreplay" (Darling, Davidson, 1986). For most women to orgasm, direct stimulation of the clitoris is necessary. When coitus has begun, there is not direct clitoral stimulation unless certain position are employed or either partner is enlightened enough to stimulate the clitoris manually. But, since manual stimulation of her clitoris during coitus is not in his best interest and she has been socialized not to touch herself, this is not likely to happen.

Therefore, it is in the best interest of the woman to try and prolong "foreplay" as long as possible. During "foreplay", the woman is more likely to receive direct clitoral stimulation from the male by way of either manual or oral stimulation. Males, following the traditional sexual script will progress from kissing thru intercourse with a period in between usually consisting of direct clitoral stimulation. Whether this type of stimulation is of her taste is uncertain. Since less than 50% of women report having an orgasm from intercourse (Hite, 1976), pre-coital activities are essential in her sexual pleasure.

Masturbation

Patriarchal beliefs become buried in the mind so they get passed onto the next generation. This is evident in parental beliefs towards masturbation. Parents tell their daughters that masturbation is wrong because someone else will satisfy their sexual needs. Also, males are socialized to believe they are in charge of female sexuality. But, the problem is created when males try to dominate an area over which they do not understand or have the ability to control.

Research shows that only 7 to 18% of parents talk to their children about masturbation (Wilson, 1975) and 40% of parents, regardless of the child's gender, say they disapprove of self-pleasuring (Roberts, et al., 1978). It has been shown that less than half of parent wanted their children to have a positive attitude toward masturbation (Gagnon, 1985). In light of the messages of the protective patriarchal ideology, the data only makes sense. One person, the female, is dependent upon the whims and desires of another, the male. He, figuratively, is always on top and in control. As for the mothers, they are seen by their male partners as being the 'good little women' for following the rules of the ideology. Interestingly enough, women who voice their thought and feelings are seen as deviant and given the title "feminists." On the other hand, traditional women try to achieve the desired title of a 'good little woman' by socializing their daughter to be passive as soon as they are born.

Passive (negative) non-verbal training generally begins when the child is an infant. If the child's hands are anywhere near her genitals, the child's hands are either removed or slapped (pain) away from her genitals. So begins the Social Circumcision of the female. The differences in the frequency of masturbation between female and males is a direct result of socialization.

In the area of masturbation, there are differences between the genders. Data shows that twice as many man than women have ever masturbated and the men that did masturbate reported three times the frequency during the same adolescent time period (Leitenberg, et al. 1993). Obviously, the same rules do not apply to males but, let us not forget who makes the rules. To Socially Circumcise males would put them on equal (sexual) footing with females and that would be definite infringement on their control.

What happens when a mother catches their daughter masturbating? These mothers, who have conformed to the 'good wife' (following, without thinking), further Socially Circumcise their daughters by spreading myths and using guilt:

> "At about eight, I made a feeble attempt at masturbation, at which I was caught by my mother, who have me a very long lecture on how this would cause me to go insane. This was my last attempt at masturbation until seven years ago, when I had my first orgasm. I am now fifty-one."
>
> "Once my mother caught me masturbating (just last year) and she was shocked, although she pretends to be enlightened and liver about sex. She told me about every part of my body except for my clitoris." (Hite, 1976, p.70)

Two Person Sexuality

In this patriarchal society, men and women are socialized to believe the male will satisfy the female's sexual needs. Males are seen as the initiators of sexual activities while females are the passive objects of male advances (Doyle, 1983).

Therefore, when females and males do come together for coitus, patriarchal scripts appear. In this country, women report they would like to reach orgasm from thrusting alone (Shotly, et al., 1984) even though other data states that less than 50% of women orgasm from intercourse (Hite, 1976). In is well known in the research that intercourse is not likely to bring about female orgasm because there is not direct clitoral stimulation. Yet, the social ideology is stronger than relevant data and is sometimes supported by data.

What is likely to happen when the woman does not orgasm from intercourse? The patriarchal script has an unwritten clause which allows blame for so-called sexual problems to fall on the shoulders of the woman. So, if the coital thrusting was long and vigorous (like the scripts says it should be), her self diagnosis may be anorgasmia—inhibited female orgasm.

There are two points that can be made of the expense of Social Circumcision and the creation of anorgasmia. First, if males were socialized differently (correctly) in relation to female sexuality, anorgasmia would not be as popular an idea. If males would stop fearing female sexuality, that could be the first step in rewriting the sexual ideology. It is always easier to blame rather that take the time to learn (in this case, unlearn).

Secondly, the frequency of anorgasmia would decrease if women were taught/allowed to learn about their sexuality and bodies. Research done by Polonko (year) revealed that 78% of women orgasmed from masturbation compared to 47% from coital thrusting. Additional research shows that of the women who masturbated, 70% reported reaching orgasm (Kinsey, 1953), 95% in Hite's Study (1976). These women who decided to go against the negative social beliefs made this discovery and found it enjoyable. Even the women who have made this discovery still battle against the sexual ideology when coming together in two person, heterosexual sex.

Data found that orgasm from masturbation is not related to female orgasm from intercourse (Fisher, 1973) because most women do not use their self-pleasuring technique during two person activities (deBruijn, 1982). Again, this falls back on the Social Circumcision of the female. She is waiting for the male to take over. It is time for women to take matters in their own hands (literally) because if the female used the same technique she used in masturbation during coital activities, she would be more likely to orgasm.

Unprepared Therapy

Since the patriarchal script is so strong, the woman may seek outside assistance to help 'cure her problem.' Seeking therapy for anorgasmia could create more problems. The therapists themselves have also been socialized by the patriarchal sexual script. Instead of looking beyond the blinders of patriarchy, the probable cause of the real problem, the therapist may insist the woman's sexual problem is mental (being fridged) or anatomical (your clitoris is not in the proper position to be stimulated by penile thrusting). It is always the woman's fault.

Today, the therapists would usually prescribe a treatment of body exploration alone or with a partner (Sensate Focus). If a woman has been socialized not to touch her genitals, this creates a problem. First, in two person sexuality, how is she supposed to tell her partner how she wants to be touched when she herself does not know? Secondly, it is not likely she will respond positively to letting someone else touch her 'down there' when she does not touch herself. The barriers of patriarchal culture have to be crossed before the woman will be able to progress to the freedom on body exploration.

The therapists must think about how this 'problem' was created and who created it. The therapists could be just as responsible, regardless of their gender, as this patriarchal culture in helping to maintain this pseudo-sexual dysfunction. The data does show that current method in treating anorgasmia are extremely successful (Reinish, 1990) but, I believe anorgasmia would not be as common if men and women were socialized correctly in relation to a woman's sexual needs and if women were more open to explore their sexuality.

The Infamous Menarche

This patriarchal society has even socialized women to be afraid of their own bodies when the topic concerns menstruation. Anything that involves the genital area gets a stigma attached to it. Since blood flows through the vagina, women are labeled hysterical, unclean and irrational. Since menstruation occurs throughout the world, these beliefs show men's fear of something they cannot do or control. As a young woman nears the time of menarche, the messages she receives are bound to affect her beliefs toward her sexuality.

Puberty in females usually beings between the ages of 8 and 13 (Gagnon, 1981) and menstruation (menarche) begins at 12.6 years of age in the United States (Udry, et al., 1986). Studies have found that mothers are the main source of information about menstruation (Logan, 1980). This is fine except for the fact that the mother has been socialized by the same patriarchal society that socialized her. The negative stories (The Curse) get passed along generation to generation thus perpetuating these cultures negative menstrual beliefs. The research states this culture has beliefs about menstrual symptoms, most negative. Such beliefs are likely to exert a powerful influence on a young woman (Clarke, Ruble, 1978). Also, if pain (cramps) accompanies her menarche, that could easily be interpreted by her that her 'forbidden area' is causing her discomfort. That is why correct information is necessary. With this inaccurate connection made, the pain will only add to her negative sexual attitude. If women were taught to look forward to these changes with the help of positive (correct) information, menstruation may be welcomed instead of feared.

If women were socialized to welcome menstruation, would body exploration start to increase? Since her body was going through such changes, exploration would enable her to become comfortable with herself as she transcends in adulthood. But, since she has been socialized for many years for the upcoming consequences of 'The Curse', the exploration is not happening.

To explain this point, I must return to masturbation. Since males receive a different version of the patriarchal script, differences appear at the ages of first masturbation. The data shows that there is a drop in the percentage of women who report their first masturbatory experience between the ages of 11 to 14 years old (Polonko, year). It is important to remember that the majority of women report these are the same years when menarche occurs. In contrast, the data shows the percentage of first masturbation in male's increases gradually with age (Clement et al., 1984). One should wonder why this same masturbation behavior (a drop in male first masturbation experience) is not evident in males when they experience nocturnal emissions? In the patriarchal script, the stigma that is associated with the genitals in not as strong for males as it is for females. Changes in the patriarchal institution must be made.

Conclusion

Since the patriarchal culture socialized women to fear their own genitals and to also depend on males for their sexual satisfaction, the patriarchal script has been shown to affect women in various areas of their well being. Males do not realize by trying to maintain their protective patriarchal world, they are putting unnecessary pressure on themselves which can only do harm in the long run. It takes an uncertain amount of energy to keep over half the worlds population oppressed. What could be achieved in this society (world) if it became an egalitarian culture and patriarchy no longer existed? Open communications, with no hidden agenda's, are necessary between the genders. Several books written about communication keeps the genders at odds with each other by saying men and women speak different languages (communicate differently). A popular book written by Dr. John Gray, "Men are from Mars, Women are from Venus", illustrate this point. It seems that Dr. Gray forgot one major point. In his eyes, men may be from Mars and women may be from Venus but, we all live here on earth! Creating a new ideology and endless open communication are the keys to success.

As I write this small but important article, I myself realize that I have also been socialized to follow the same patriarchal script. Whenever you read, you must always read between the words themselves. Patriarchy teaches that heterosexuality is natural, which I did follow blindly throughout this article. People who are gay follow their own social script. This causes fear (homophobia) because the traditional society cannot cast their influence over them. That is one of the reasons why gays and lesbians are seen as abnormal. Even thought, I am in the twenty-plus age group, I have a lot of un-learning ahead of me.

12

Sex and the Listserv

Let's start from the basics. A listserv is many people discussing various topics through in internet. Even though there are many types of "e-conferences" (Usenet, alt.groups, etc.) they all share the same goal. Listservs connect people who have similar interest and it allows them to communicate to each other.

Behind the scenes of a listserv is the list-owner or moderator. Some moderators run a hands-off list with others are extremely hands-on while they 'police' the information that comes across their list. Some moderators run un-moderated lists, in letting every post get forwarded to the member list without review. Other moderators run list that are constantly reviewed, checking every post to see if it is on topic or not. With full moderation, if the post is not on topic, it will be deleted by the moderator and never reach the list (Robinson, 1996).

Since we live in an electronic age, many educators/professors have incorporated the internet use into their curricula. Early on, professors used e-mail which they quickly discovered became a problem, especially if they had a large class. First, the students did not give their own e-mail address. They felt they could use a friend's e-mail address. The problem was those accounts were not checked regularly to keep up with assignments. Secondly, some students had e-mail accounts through ISPs with missing identifying information. That could become problematic for the professor who tries to verify student participation and/or sending individual e-mail messages. Third, keeping a mailing list can be time consuming. Student may change their e-mail address several times during the semester. To add, those students who changed their e-mail address could become upset with the professor for not knowing they had actually changed their address. Fourth, in using an e-mail mailing list, the same question could be asked over and over again. Even if the professor saves the answer, they will still end up with a large amount of time being wasted.

In using a listserv, much of the 'weight' gets shifted from the professor to the student. The student is responsible for subscribing to the list. If there are any issues with joining the list, the student has to make the corrections and reapply until their subscription is complete. To add, the student is responsible for keeping their address current on the listserv. They will have to unsubscribe and re-subscribe using their new address. Also, when students receive a mailing, they have to options to (a) lurk and observe the discussion, (b) respond to the listserv where everyone can see their thoughts or, (c) respond directly to the individual who wrote the original posting (Overbaugh, 1998).

How else are teachers and students using listservs to communicate with each other? In 1997, Don Leu created the RTEACHER listserv to give educators the chance to discuss literacy education. Over the past 6-years, RTEACHER now has approximately 1,200 subscribers all over the globe. This listserv seems to thrive on conversations that are important to the well-being of literacy education (Brabham & Villaume, 2003). Many of these listserv discussions have focused on the ways to provide practice as they helped students apply strategies used by skillful readers. The postings to the listserv described how teachers used strategies such as questioning, making connections, visualizing, inferring summarizing, and synthesizing. The teachers posted how excited they were when their strategies resulted in more "strategic and thoughtful reading in [their] students" (Villaume & Brabham, 2002, p.672).

Also, there is another group of elementary school teachers who are linked through a listserv. This listserv is called the Teachers Networking Together (TNT) which is sponsored by the Exxon Education

Foundation. These teachers introduced a program called My Make-Believe Castle to their students. This program incorporates three modes of problem solving; (1) pointing and clicking, (2) wandering and wondering, and (3) persistent probing. The listserv allows the teachers to share their students' problem-solving abilities with other teachers. Also, My Make-Believe Castle has evolved into a research project. The teachers introduce the program to their students, and with little intervention, the teachers monitor their students actions, conversations and decisions they made while playing the game. As the original teachers began to share the comments and questions through the listserv, more and more teachers became interested in My Make-Believe Castle (Martin & Bearden, 1998).

One of the most important aspects of using a listserv is deciding if this listserv is for you. An important issue is whether or not the topic of the moment is important to you right now. The topics in listservs are known to change overtime. Therefore, your decision to remain a member of the listserv is an on-going process. A listserv that had important information when you initially joined may change into something that is not helpful to you. Some issues you can use to evaluate a listserv are:

1. Does the information from the listserv have value to me?

2. Do I have the time necessary to deal with all the new mail from the listserv?

3. Do the discussions stay on or close to the initial topic?

4. Is the information accurate?

5. Do the members of the conversation seem to be knowledgeable regarding the topic? (Robinson, 1996).

It's been said that using listservs can be confusing and frustrating. There can be a fair amount of problems but there can be benefits as well. It is important to explore and be patient. First, make sure you subscribe to groups that you have an interest in. This is where using an on-line search tool can come in handy. If they are not what you want then, unsubscribe and try something else. If the listservs' topics are fine but the mail is too much, contact the moderator for information on how to receive mail using the digest format. After all, it is important not to feel overwhelmed (Robinson, 1996).

In my own searches for a good listserv, I ran into several problems. I will expand on these later in this paper. To being, I had to join three listservs in the hope of finding something of interest. The first one I joined was a sexuality listserv through the University of Washington. They have a rather large website called sexuality.org. It is a fairly well known site, especially for those of us who are in the field of sexuality. On the subscribe page, there was a few lines concerning the amount of letters one would received if they joined the site. I was warned of getting around 500 messages per day. Well, after I subscribed, I had to wait a few days for my first letter to arrive. I subscribed in digest form but, many of my early letters were just other members inquiring whether this list was still active. It took awhile but the letters started to appear. Some letters were still a waste of time but that tends to happen with an unmoderated listserv.

The other two lists I joined were of little use to me. I joined another list that is located at Texas A&M University. This list is also about sex and sexuality. I really did stumble across this list. This list arrived fairly consistently but, the conversations were really juvenile and had little substance to me. Using my own criteria, I felt like the members of this group were all horny undergraduates who were more interested in asking questions for their shock value alone. Not my style ... maybe ten years ago but definitely not now.

The third and final list I joined was called HEDIR (). This was a health education listserv. I actually wrote to the moderator and he have me the heads up about the list (actually, I wrote to a professor of mine and she told me about the list. She also told me about the list she belongs to {AASECT—the American Association for Sex Education, Counselors and Therapists} but, I did not have the $100 required to join and become a member of their list. I am sure that list has all of the sexual heavyweights on it and I am fairly sure their discussions are interesting. I will join it later. Anyhow, the HEDIR list was rather dry for my tastes. Every so often, a posting would appear regarding new research from the CDC or National Institutes of Health. There were plenty of job posting and a few questions from people looking for information about an issue (healthy living, stress, new textbooks, etc). I am not saying this information was not important, it was not for me. After all, it was a health education site and not a sexuality site which I had a definite preference for. This is why I chose to focus on the listserv from the sexuality.org. It was more what I wanted but, it still had its share of problems.

The moderator of this list is Dan Lyke. He seems to keep this list fairly unmoderated. Eventhough this list is about sex and sexuality, I received a single item digest. It was a question regarding what one would do if they won a billion dollars (the Pepsi-Cola promotion). He let it pass through and only a few people responded to that post. Dan seemed to appear when the list was having problems or people were not unsubscribing correctly. He would say his few words and vanish into the background again. He seems to like it that way.

No one (who I saw) identified as an actual sexuality professional. No one really talked about have a degree or where they worked. It seems many of the members are sex experts in their own way. Some of the members discussed their own sexual behaviors down to the last detail. Several talked about belonging to the S&M community. Whenever someone mentioned S&M, they would appear. It was nothing major though. Some of the major topics included circumcision, movies, positive sexuality, S&M, sex in the workplace, and just general sex. I got the feeling these people were fairly liberal in their sexual attitudes, behaviors and opinions. Many of the members posting were based on their opinion which was rarely supported by citing research or where they heard the information. It was like some of them read *a* sexuality textbook and along with their own sexual activities, decided they are knowledgeable enough and have no problem in giving their opinion. There were two discussions I decided to follow. My favorite was started by a girl {who said she was 18 years old}. The members discussed her opinions and I felt had a really productive chat. I will write a bit more about this conversation later.

To add, since some of the members liked to give their opinion, a few of them seemed like they really enjoyed being the center of attention. They would post over and over again. I got the feeling they were trying to become 'net-famous' and use their 15-minutes of fame on this listserv. For me, the example of this is a person named Jonathan. When I joined the list, he was involved in a discussion about circumcision. He would write these really long posts. Then, when some would reply, he would say they did not understand what he was saying and make it personal. There were a few people who tried to have a discussion with him but it was to no avail. {I actually started to get tired of the guy! When I was reading his posts, I got to the point where I would just ignore what he had to say}.

Sex in the work place

One of the topics from this listserv was called Sex in the Work place. This topic was only discussed a few times (from what I saw). I focused on this topic just because of the whole sexual harassment angle. One writer actually mentioned how she was assaulted by her boss. This is one of the first posts where I came across Jonathan.

1. Jonathan writes:
    On a related note I do wish that we could have more sex in the work place here, and grabbing of buttocks and crotches. The French reportedly look at us with disgust in this regard, and rightly so. It's time IMO to bring more sex and nudity into the work place. We ought to be able to IMO wear a little sign or button at work which means "yes, you can grab mine if you want."

2. Rosa responded:
    We can have sex in the work place, simply must be consensual and possibly discreet. What we can't have is inappropriate grab-

bing of buttocks and crotches. I guess you've never been a backed into a corner by a very attractive person, who happens to be your boss and demands a kiss while fondling your breasts (or penis or ass). From personal experience its not lots of fun ... you come away doubting yourself and wondering what is wrong with you for feeling like you've been violated by this person who others dream about. It has nothing to do with sexual hang-ups, prudish beliefs or repression. It is about consent to allow whom you want to touch you to do so pleasurably and for those you do not want to touch you to respect your wishes and personal boundaries.

3. Jonathan responded with:
    I can see that we're getting along nicely here. Relative to my posi-tion your statement is largely non-sequitur. However I'm also glad that you did not omit my statement, which I shall quote again: "We ought to be able to IMO wear a little sign or button at work which means 'yes, you can grab mine if you want.'"

Circumcision

Though the life of the listserv, this was one of the larger discussions. It went on for days and days. Once again, Jonathan was in the middle of the discussion. I will admit early on to reading this discussion but after awhile, it was extremely boring and dry. Yes, I do agree the issue of circumcision/genital mutilation is important but, I wrote about this topic over ten years ago and I have since, as a person, moved on.

1. Jonathan said:
    Perhaps some people may find mutilated bodies more attractive than mutilated ones. So be it. I can have my opinion about such people. If a person was circed they have to live with it, or attempt partial restoration, but on the whole IMO a whole penis is more beautiful than a mutilated one. And I say that as someone with a mutilated one. I still find my penis beautiful at times, but it's not as beautiful as if it were whole and untouched by the hands of thoughtless butchers.

2. Joe Dial said:

   If you want to rail against circ because it's done on unconsenting babies, go to. But when you tell someone they are wrong for their sense of what is attractive or not, when you question their sanity for preferring a body modification, you're doing to them exactly what the majority culture does to you when the question is your own sexual tastes and activities Sexual mutilations are always done by dominator societies and the purpose is always to control. When we circumcise males, their brains are encoded with violence to a part of the body that is meant to experience pleasure. Pain and pleasure are confused. Rage is instilled. It is not surprising that the most violent people in the world are the Muslims, Jews, and North Americans. Violence inflicted on infants and children creates violent beings.

I decided to cut of this posting right here. There are so many, I just gave up. Then in some of the later postings, it seems like Jonathan gets personal or takes opinions personal and the discussion seems to spin out of control. I just felt it was important to mention this discussion in the paper because it was a large discussion.

<u>Butt Watching</u>

For me, this had to be one of the more entertaining posts. In today's climate of sexual harassment, I am surprised someone would dare even to mention this. But, since there are no faces on this site, I guess people feel it is ok to hide behind their computer screen. As a sexuality educator, I can understand both sides of the argument. The responses from the initial posts are from women (I think) and are quite honest and open minded.

1. Amit S wrote:

   Hi all, OK call me a pervert but I like watching women's derrières. Why do women, in this age of equality, object to such behavior. I am sure a man wouldn't mind it if a women were to do that to him. I wonder what the women here think of this.

2. Amy Russo responded with:
    Good Morning Amit! Speaking for myself, I have no problem
    with a man looking at my butt. My lover enjoys looking every
    chance he gets, as well as making appreciative comments when I
    bend over. Knowing that he finds that area attractive is a turn on
    to me. And yes, I love to look at not only his butt, but I look
    while out and about, too. Have a great day!

3. Joanne responded with:
    A lot of women dress to call attention to themselves; me
    included. Sure, we all like to look nice, and if it pleases someone
    else and they get pleasure from watching us, we both win. As for
    eyeing our rears, I like to think mine is well shaped and if a guy is
    attracted to it, that's fine with me, as long as he doesn't press up
    against it on a crowded bus or subway.
    Joanne S.

I wish this discussion was larger than the few posts it received. This
is one of the things about listservs I do not like. The discussions I
could care less about are long and overblown. This topic was nice and
fun while the women who responded (I think they were women) were
open and honest. Lets be honest, I know many men who take a peek
at a woman's tush. I also know many women who look at guys bot-
toms as well. At least these people were honest about it.

Good Information

I think overall, this was my favorite discussion. It was nice but at the
same time, I was a bit concerned. This posting was started by a young
woman who said she was 18 years old. Now, in some parts of the
country, this would be illegal and people could get in trouble. Also, I
think sometime there are police/federal officers on the net who post a
kids to trap adults who have no harmful motives. Yes, this does happen. In digest 2512, she posted many times in a row. For some reason, this looks like a trap—like the authorities were putting out bait
to see who would bite. Anyhow, this woman asked good questions

while the members of the group responded to her in a helpful, non-predator manner. Well, at least I see it that way. Here is what they said.

1. Krista G. wrote:
    Isn't the orgasm the highest point of sexual relations physiologically? If you can't have an orgasm, then you haven't had the physiologically ultimate sexual encounter, have you? You may have had a wonderful experience in all other respects, but in terms of sex, you haven't completed.

2. In reply to Krista G, Ron wrote:
    In direct answer to your question, no orgasm is not "the highest point of sexual relations." Here's the shocker, there is no absolute "highest point" in sexual relations. There is no objective standard by which to compare yourself to and figure out if you're as high as you can go. In fact, the entire concept of "high" doesn't really work here. :)

3. In a very nice (extremely long) reply, Dodger wrote:
    >*Isn't the orgasm the highest point of sexual relations physiologically?*
    Depends how you're defining "highest point". Some might call it the *conclusion* of sexual "relations" (another term that needs definition, if we're going to have a precise analysis), but I'd say that's quite open for debate as well.
    >*If you can't have an orgasm, then you haven't had the physiologically ultimate sexual encounter, have you?* Again, you're assigning emotional baselines to what is a physical act. ("highest point", "ultimate", etc.) Shouldn't you be the one deciding what the highest point of any activity is for you? Let's say several people climb a mountain. Ask them all what the highest point of the exercise was. You're likely to get several different answers: Standing at the peak and looking for miles, coming back down, making that last push for the summit, crossing the crevasse, watching the eagle soar by, etc.

<However, if partners constantly rely on fantasy or a BDSM scene to get off, how are they having a romantic sexual relationship? I can't answer that for two reasons: 1) I can't speak for what goes on in anybody else's mind. I have no idea what they consider romantic, or why. And, 2) I don't associate sexual activity with romance. Romance is romance and sex is sex. You can have both together or you can have them separate (yes, even with the same person), but in and of themselves they are completely independent of one another.*

Here, this is were the listserv seemed to shine. The posts really seemed to have some thought behind them with out the posturing I observed in some of the other discussions. Plus, I agreed with what the posters had to say. Of course, it is easy to agree with something that you have an affection for—positive sexual health. In these posts, I felt the authors had experience in what they were talking about. Maybe, they were educated in sexuality through personal experience or held open opinions and gained their information through books. Also, the fact there was little profanity/smut in the post showed me these members were more about the education versus the shock value of words. Do not get me wrong, there were some posts on the listserv that got me hot under the collar but, for the most part, this discussion was professional.

Doing this paper was a bit frustrating for me. I had to join several lists just to get information. A few of the lists reported having over 100 posts per day but, they never really appeared. It was depressing after awhile. Then, with out warning, all of the lists started to run and I was getting to many letters. Then, I had to weed through them and I discovered many of the postings were just junk and of little use to me. That is why I ended up staying with the sexuality listserv. It was in my field of interest and I receiving posts on a regular basis.

I started my own group a few years ago. I only had a few members and topica.com finally shut it down a few months ago. In total, I think it received 10 postings in 4 years of existence. It was a sexual health listserv (I started a special interest group inside my national sexuality organization—the Society for the Scientific Study of Sexuality (SSSS). They have a web site as well. I may create another listserv later on.

Hey, I just had an idea. Since I just spent the last semester creating a sexuality web site, I was wondering if you could tell me if Widener has the ability to host and support listserves? I know other schools have them. I think a sexuality listserv here at Widener would be a nice book end for my web site. Any thoughts? See you around.

Hot

Ok ... officially my paper has ended. Just as I said earlier, there are some posting that are explicit. That listserv is definately for adults. After much deliberation, I decided to copy one of the *tamer* postings from the listserv. **WARNING**—He does not hold back. Good luck!

1. Also, it takes time for a couple to attune to each other. A few years ago I moved in with a woman who had to have her cunt licked for a long time before she'd cum. A year later I would still lick her cunt for ages but she'd just cum successively every few minutes the whole time. She never ever did get off on missionary sex without manual clitoral stimulation but paradoxically did cum once when we were having anal sex at the same time I did. We became so well attuned that we could have mutual oral sex during which she'd cum 3 or 4 times the last being when I came in her mouth. I'd continue on her and she'd cum again straight away. She was a very keen masturbator and the more sex we'd have at night the more she would Jill-off in the morning. At one stage we went for a few months just wanking {masturbate}in each other's company and it was excellent sex. The last year we were together we just did not bother with penile/vaginal sex, the other stuff we did was far more satisfactory.

13

Swingers

One of the best arguments against an exclusive relationship is from Freud. In a paper on the "Civilized Sexual Morality and Modern Nervous Illness," he downplayed the requirement of no sexual intercourse outside of marriage, which he argues could lead to a nervous illness. Freud (1908) was particularly worried about the high frequency of impotence in men and frigidity in women, as well as the way the inhibition of sexual curiosity in women scared them away from any form of knowledge.

In 1912, Freud discussed the question of whether this happened because of the natural instinct or the control civilization placed on love and sensual pleasures. He said:

> "The fact that the curb put upon love by civilization involves a universal tendency to debase sexual objects will perhaps lead us to turn our attention from the object to the instincts themselves. The damage caused ... is seen in the fact that the freedom later given to that pleasure in marriage does not bring full satisfaction. But at the same time, if sexual freedom is unrestricted from the outset the result is not better." (Freud, 1912, p.187)

An open marriage was originally defined as a non-manipulative relationship of peers with role flexibility in which was no need for dominance and submission, or for stifling possessiveness (O'Neill & O'Neill, 1972). With regard to extramarital sex, the O'Neill's considered this a person's choice, especially when the couple has sufficient trust, identity, and open communication. What was new in the O'Neill's definition of marriage was that it put honesty and commitment above all else, including sexual fidelity.

To continue, the O'Neill's (1974) felt in today's society, people are not educated for marriage or in the requisites of a good human relationship, nor are they aware of the psychological and the dozens of other commitments that they typical marriage contract implies. The expectations of the closed marriage—the major one being that one partner will be able to fulfill all of the other's needs (emotional, social, sexual, economic, intellectual, and otherwise)—present obstacles to growth and attitudes that foster conflict between partners. In a1973 interview with George O'Neill, he commented on the current practice of marriage:

> "This whole business of legal, traditional, old fashioned, closed marriage—the way it has been in America for the last 200 years—is being rejected by a lot of people ... Besides, closed marriage is just as much an ideal model as is open marriage, and most couple fit in somewhere between the two. (p.18)

In an interview with Nena O'Neill, she refers to *The Marriage Premise* (O'Neill, 1977), where she feels the traditional ideals of commitment and sharing are affirmed and in which equality was presented as a support for sexual fidelity. She says,

> "We thought that a couple who had already developed that ... emotionally secure and strong primary relationship ... would be able to deal with the issue of sex outside their marriage. Based on our research, we also felt that open and honest discussion of desires and fantasies would defuse desires and minimize jealousy ... (p.203).

In contrast to open marriages, there is another label called swinging. Bartell (1971) says the term "swinger" is the name used to denote the people who participate as a couple in sexual relations with at least one other individual, and it implies an avant-garde and free life style.

Becoming a Swinger

In most cases, it is the men who bring up the idea of swinging which was usually met with a negative reaction by the woman. One study found that 68% of the males made the initial suggestion to swing. The males alone made 59% of all final decisions to swing; 28% were joint decision to swing and only 12% of the women made the final decision to swing (Henshel, 1973). The typical reaction from the woman was that something was wrong with her marriage, followed by a strong hatred for the whole idea. At this point, the man usually beings a "convincing process" which was done to ease her fears (Varni, 1974).

It appears there was a time lapse between the time the couples learned about swinging and the time when they considered it more seriously. More time passed before the final decision was reached, indicating that the decision making here was multiphasic (Safilios-Rothschild, 1970). Unfortunately in the Henshel (1973) study, her participants could not remember well enough the duration of the various time spans involved.

According to Varni (1974), he says there are two conditions that have to be present together in order to be a swinger. First, the couple engages in extramarital sex with full knowledge and consent of one another. There is no lying or cheating involved. Second, the couple engages in extramarital sex together. The fact they do it together establishes a necessary condition of swinging. Because the couple engages in extramarital sex with the full knowledge of their partner, they do not view themselves as adulterers. In contrast, they view themselves of having transcended the immaturity and dishonesty of affairs engaged in by other couples. Therefore, the swingers are able to turn the deviant label around and apply it to those non-swinging couples who engage in extramarital sex.

There are two factors that are important for a woman to become fond of swinging. They are 1) her perception of her marriage relationship and 2) her own subjective experience. If the woman feels her relationship has not been damaged, she is relieved. If she feels the relationship has been improved, she is pleased. If her subjective experience was not negative, she is relieved. If it was at all a positive experience, she is pleased.

Earlier on in her swinging, women are usually more concerned with the stability of their relationships. When she feels her relationship is not threatened, her subjective feeling take preference. The same two factors are present for the men as well. For men, it seems importance is attached to both factors for having a favorable experience. It is important to remember the men have a vested interest in their partners' having a positive experience, since their continued swinging is depended on her participation.

If nothing tragic happens during their first experience, the couple is likely to try it again. The second experience is usually more enjoyable since the couple has a better understanding of what is takes place. Because of their prior experience, their anxiety levels are lower and they are able to relax and enjoy themselves. If nothing negative happens during the second experience, especially if it is enjoyable, it is usually the clincher and it validates the 'non-uniqueness' of the first experience.

If a couple decides they will not swing anymore, it is usually because of unmanageable jealousy on the part of either the husband or wife, or sometimes both. Most swingers agree that the preconditions for having a successful swinging life are 1) the couples' relationship is based on love; 2) each person has no serious hang-up's; and 3) there should be no jealously (Varni, 1974).

Types of Swingers

According to Gilmartin (1975), there are different types of swingers. At one end of a continuum, there are purely sexual swingers who desire no social or emotional relationships with their partners. At the other end, there are swingers who desire close and lasting relationships or friendships. In the middle are the 'recreational swingers', who usually belong to swinging clubs with stable and limited memberships, and who consider the social aspects of swinging almost as important as the sexual.

Charles Varni (1974) defined the types of swingers even further than Gilmartin. Varni divided the swingers into five categories:

1. *Hard-core*: These swingers do not want any emotional involvement with their partners, have little selectivity of partners and usually swing with as many couples as possible. They are said to be cold, unfeeling, and deviant by other types of swingers. In the hard-core couple, the woman is usually coerced into swinging. They are also known to participate in unstable party and one-couple situations.

2. *Egotistical*: These swingers do not want an emotional involvement with their partners and are usually selective of their sexual partners. They want the sexual experience and seek to gratify their own sexual needs and desires, which may involve feeling attractive, virile, sexy and desired buy other persons. Swinging is viewed as a separate part of their lives and they have few social relationships with their swinging partners. They tend to enjoy party and one-couple situations.

3. *Recreational*: These swingers focus on the social aspects that go along with swinging. They are members of fairly stable groups, enjoy party and one-couple situations. Swinging is viewed as an entertaining social activity where a strong emotional attachment to the partner is neither needed nor desired.

4. *Interpersonal*: They desire and focus on the close emotional relationships with their partners. They seek intimate and viable friendships with their partners. The sex aspect fulfills and completes their relationship and their life experience. The couple

views swinging as a natural part of their lifestyle. They are very selective with whom they swing and prefer one-couple situations exclusively, and many of their friends will be swingers.

5. *Communal:* They are similar to *interpersonal* but, they support some form of group marriage, an idea that is rejected by almost all other swingers.

Characteristics of Swingers

The research has found that the majority of swingers fall into the middle and upper middle classes. They have also found swingers tend to have an above average education (Gilmartin, 1975; Jenks, 1985b; Levitt, 1988) and income (Jenks, 1985b; Levitt, 1988) and tend to work in the professional and/management positions (Jenks, 1985b; Levitt, 1988).

Studies have shown that the majority (over 90%) of swingers are white. The mean age in the Levitt study was 40.7 and in the Bartell study, the majority clustered in the 28-34 age group.

Politically, swingers reported they were moderate to conservative and identify with the Republican Party. While 50% voted for Ronald Reagan in 1980, only 23.7% voted for Carter (Jenks, 1986). Further, it has been found (Flanigan and Zingale, 1991) that people with higher income and higher education tend to vote Republican. From the reported prior research, swingers tend to have above average incomes and education. Therefore, swingers could be voting for their social class interests.

The one area where swingers seem to be liberal is in the area of sexuality. A study involving 400 swingers found they were significantly more liberal than a control group of non-swingers. The swingers were especially more liberal in areas such as divorce, premarital sex, pornography, homosexuality and abortion (Jenks, 1985a).

A study by Bartell (1970) reported that the majority of his sample did not attend church regularly. The Jenks' (1985b) study found that sixty-six percent of his sample did not have any religious affiliation.

These numbers are consistent with other studies which showed sixty-three percent did not have any religious affiliation (Gilmartin, 1975). What is interesting is that even though 70% said they did not currently attend church services, many said they attended church every week when they were growing up. So, it seems many swingers were raised in religious homes but they gave up their religion on their way to adulthood. This is in direct contrast to the American population where 92% claim a religious preference (Gallup & Castelli, 1989) and only 4% said they were "totally non-religious" (Bezilla, 1993).

Gilmartin (1975) found that the swinger's parents, especially for the males, did not subject them to many rules or regulations. In the face of their freedom, many swingers felt they were held down by parental control than the non-swingers during their teenage years. So, even with few rules, the swingers felt a greater need for independence than non-swingers.

Gediman (1975) felt that people who were creative require a variety in the stimulus and/or in their love object. She sited Greenacre et al. on the possibility that specially gifted people may have "an unusual sensitivity to all sensory and kinesthetic stimulation". (p.421). Therefore, it may be possible this idea may be appropriate to the observation that a number of intelligent and creative people are drawn to experimentation with sexually open relationships.

Perceptions of Swingers

It seems that swingers are not viewed as the highest standing citizens in our society. Gilmartin (1975) found around fifty percent of non-swingers would mind if an "otherwise unobjectionable swinging couple moved into their neighborhood" (p.55). What is even better is the fact that many of the people in his research had neighbors who were swingers. Gilmartin said, "However hypothetical this situation may have seemed to the controls, each of them did in fact have swingers neighbors." He continues, "I had selected each control couple mainly on this basis of their proximity to a swinging couple, usually within the same block." (p.55)

To go even deeper, Jenks (1985b) did a study with 100 non-swingers to give their opinions about swingers. Jenks then compared their answers to over 300 who were also involved in the study. The swingers were perceived as using alcohol, smoking marijuana and other drugs far more than the swingers themselves stated. To add, the non-swingers overestimated the number of non-whites who participated in swinging, on having a liberal philosophy, and political affiliation. When asked to compare attitudes, the non-swingers placed themselves away from where they though the swingers be. Also, more that fifty—percent of the non-swingers felt that the swingers were in need of therapy where only 26% of the swingers had been in therapy.

Reasons for Swinging

Why do people enter into swinging? What caused them to become involved in an activity that is clearly outside of the mainstream in this society? Research has found a number of reasons why.

One of the main reasons for getting involved in swinging is for the variety of partners and sexual experiences. When asked what was your main reason for swinging, one study found that 'variety' was named (Jenks, 1986).

Jenks (1986) found the second most popular reason given was for the pleasure or excitement. Also included in this was the idea of the 'forbidden fruit'—given the chance to participate in a deviant lifestyle and to defy social norms.

Bartell (1970) found another reason for swinging was for the increased social life. The possibility of meeting new people was found to be very important with this study sample.

Also in the Bartell (1970) study, he found watching others perform gave them the chance to observe new sexual techniques. The swingers would then use the new techniques when they returned to their marital relationship or to overcome any sexual inhibitions, which they may have had with their partner.

Stinnett & Birdsong (1978) found some other reasons given for swinging. They found swinging gave some people the chance to recapture their youth, to provide an ego lift for the person in that they learn they are still attractive and desirable to others, and their sexual interest in their partner increases.

Even though, the husbands seem to have the advantage in decision making about swinging, it is the women who tend to adapt better to the new sexual freedom than their husbands. The women may obtain more sexual gratification than their husbands and swinging may be an important channel of socialization toward true sexual freedom for them. For example, sexual freedom and equality is seen as an improvement over the double standard and one could conclude that is a good thing. If this is true, the women's improvement in their sexual freedom could off set their decision-making disadvantage and could be valued higher than any possible advantage gained if they were the decision makers (Henshel, 1973).

Effects on Marriage

Swinging does not to appear to have any negative effects on marriages. About 85% of both husbands and wives feel swinging posed no threat to their marriages, or to their love for their spouses. In this study, no one felt their marriage has become worse since they began to swing. The great majority of husbands and wives felt their marriage has improved. When swingers rated their marriages compared to non-swingers, the swingers especially the husbands, were found to have a higher level of marital satisfaction and adjustment (Gilmartin, 1975).

More than half of the swinging couples have sex together more than four time a week, compared to only 16% of the non-swinging couples. Many of the swingers reported that rather than dampening their passion for each other, their swinging adventures often caused an increase in sexual interest. Many of the swingers had sex together immediately after returning home from a swinging party. Moralists and social commentators have described swingers as unhappy, undisciplined, bored, neurotic or perverted. In his research, Gilmartin (1975) says he "found no evidence to support such assumptions." (p.58)

Does sexual openness cause jealously? And, does not jealously break up the marriage? Another study found their participants were remarkably free from jealously. When jealousy did become a serious problem, the couples did not break up but chose to stop having sex outside of the marriage (or, in some cases, to stop being open about it). Jealousy was hardly even the reason given for a break up.

The same study looked at the patterns for entering in to swinging. They observed many of the couples began with closed marriages and over time, changed to an open relationship. In this study, none of the couples started with an open relationship and changed to closed. Of the few open relationships that failed, it is important to remember they all started out as closed relationships and were changed afterwards. The author felt, because of the negative social pressure, it is unwise to label those relationships as a failed open marriage because the closed marriage came before the open marriage (Rubin & Adams, 1986).

Denfeld (1974) said when a couple is "not emotionally capable" or "the primary relationship bond either was not solidified first or was neglected" and the couple initiated an open relationship to "save the marriage," the effort usually failed (Knapp & Whitehurst, 1977, p.151). Some 'failures' of open marriages are in fact 'failures' to restore an already problematic closed marriage. This is an important item to remember when comparing closed versus open marriages.

Conclusion

I have to say this is been one of the most informative papers I have ever written. I actually had fun while I was writing. I never knew there was so much that went on when a couple decides to start to swing. For some reason, I was under the impression it was something couples did when they wanted to spice up their bedroom. I had a feeling after a couple "swung" a few times together, they would become friends. I'm wondering about the swingers who just have sex and leave, with no desire for further contact. Yes, some people can withdraw the emotional aspect of the sexuality from their behavior but, that's tough for me to accept. Yes, there are some people who view sexuality just as a body function and nothing more. For me, I'm not sure I could do that. It just seems kind of cold.

The big question for me is could I be a swinger? If I was able to swing as a single guy, yes but I would still be very particular. I'm particular now, almost to the point of being insane. If I was married, I'm not sure. Right now, I would say yes but with conditions. I would say yes but my wife could only swing with other females and me. (God, sounds so traditional; that whole insecure male thing!). I'm just trying to imagine what I would think if I looked over and I saw my wife being totally worked over by some other guy. Since I have never been in that situation before, I cannot say how I would react but right now, I don't think it would be too pleasant.

I have to say thanks to the Internet, I was able to do some exploring. I came across an organization called the NASCA. It is an organization that is dedicated to the promotion of the swinging lifestyle. According to their web site [www.nasca.com], their international conference claims to have been attended by over 40,000 people. Why is it they get 40,000 people and SSSS is lucky to get 400? How interesting is that?

I also came across a web site called Freedom Acres. It is another on-premises swinger club located in California. On their site, they say:

> "The club offers a very open atmosphere of sexuality, you can expect to see partial nudity, full nudity as well as sexual activity almost anywhere in the club. Each couple is free to become as involved as they are comfortable with. It is a very low pressure atmosphere and ideal for couples just beginning their adventures into this lifestyle." [www2.freedomacres.com]

Well, I have to tell you I did some more digging and I came across a few swingers clubs in the local area. I actually found one in Philadelphia. Its called Club Kama Sutra. [www.clubkamasutra.com] They have parties on Friday night. It costs $75 per couple, $5 for single ladies, and $80 for single guys. On Saturday, its $15 for single women and single men are not allowed.

On the Internet, the site shows pictures of the club and it looks pretty upscale. The club looks nice and clean with a fairly large dance floor. The site says, on the first floor, there is a full dinner with a new menu every week. Dinner starts at 10pm and breakfast is served at 1am. I guess the second floor is where all the fun stuff takes place. There are a couple of lounges and all of the ceilings have mirrors on them. They even have showers, towels and toiletries.

Now, after seeing the pictures on the Internet, I am dying to go see what Club Kama Sutra is all about. If I wanted to get in, I would guess I would have to find someone to fake it. Since I am single, I may have to ask one a few friends of mine if they would be interested in going to a swingers club with me. I do not plan on participating with any of the 'players'. I'm more interested in trying to absorb the atmosphere of the club. I would like to make a few observations on the clientele who go to the club. If anyone approaches me to 'join in', I would just tell them I'm not interested.

Finally, I must say I learned so much more about swinging than I ever thought I would learn. I've always heard rumors and crazy stories about swingers. Now, I understand that they are just regular folks just like the rest of us. I can't say I was biased for or against them, I just wanted to learn more information about them. So I did!

Epilogue:
My Sexual History

(Names have been changed)

Boy, oh boy. This is going to be interesting. When I used to teach at CUNY, my students had a choice of either going to a sex boutique, going to a gay/lesbian club or writing a sexual history. Of course, there were several students who used to write their sexual histories. Now, I am a student again and I have to write one. Talk about fair play.

I can only remember a few things about my sexual education when I was growing up. I can remember a few things in vivid detail and other things are blurred or totally blocked. On the 2nd day of class, I was talking to "Sharon" about trying to remember things I did when I was little that added to my sex education. We came to the consensus that there were just some items that are just gone because they are just too buried under the years of everything else called life. Well, here is what I could remember.

This one is pretty clear. I remember one day my mother sending me upstairs to get the broom from their room. It was dark so I asked her where it was. She told me it was behind the door. When I looked behind the door and I saw the broom and I saw something else as well. There was a poster of sexual positions on the back of the door. What was cool was the fact that the positions glowed in the dark, neon green I do believe. I just remember looking up at this poster and comprehending the importance of this poster. I was thinking 'well, it must be important because it's glowing at me.' After a few minutes, I actually took the broom down stairs and gave it to my mom.

Several months after that, my friends and I played Truth or Dare. This is the story I told in class about being the first to have "sex". Still, I wonder what in my brain caused me to offer to do it. I'm still fascinated by my definition of sex at that time. Where did that develop? I know I was under 5 years old and from someplace, I developed a concept of sex. I could have walked in on my parents or something but how would I have known to define their behavior as sex at such a young age? My best guess is that I did walk in on them and their response (yelling, screaming for me to get out, or something) could have told me their activity was important in some way and it was important enough to be put away in my brain.

But, what I don't understand is the way I had "sex" with that young girl. We were just standing there, tummy to tummy, not moving or anything. How did I know even to do that? Where did that information come from? If anything, one would think we should have been lying down. There is something there I no longer have access too. I've been trying to remember for the longest time, ever since you gave us this assignment. It's just too far gone!

Next came kindergarten. For this, I had to be around 5 or 6 years old. There was a girl named "Susan" who used to pull her pants down and run around. I thought Susan was cool so I hung around her a lot. At my old school, we used to go places and hide and I used to hide with Susan. She showed me her vulva way back then. I even have a slight memory of the scent of baby powder. I know she let me touch it because the baby powder smell was on my fingers.

Then, in the first grade, my teacher's husband built us a small playhouse. It was just big enough for 2 people. So, we turned that house into a kissing booth. We used to take turns going into the booth and kissing whoever. I do believe that all of my choices were female. There were two windows on the side and people used to stand with their back against them for privacy. I do remember I also had a few girlfriends in the first grade. One of their names was "Tiffany". I remember this because I bought her a gift for x-mas one year and my mom drove me to her house so I could give it too her.

I skipped 2nd grade and in the 3rd grade, and I met "Sue." She was a blue-eyed blond who was really cute. We used to sneak away at school and kiss. This was about the time when I started to really play doctor. She used to let me explore everything. Those were the good old days. At my old school, we used to go on camping trips and of course, we used to sneak away all the time.

At 4th grade, I changed schools and I hated it. In 5th grade, I went back to my old school. That was when I met "Dawn." She was my girlfriend and a serious one at that. Our teacher used to read to the class. Dawn and I used to sit under a table and fondle each other. She had her hand down my pants and I had my hand in hers. Everyone in class knew what was going on. I swear the teacher knew but didn't care.

It was during a school camping that I received my first blowjob. There were two couples, Dawn and I and my best friend and his girlfriend. Dawn and I had talked about it before and she said ok. Still there was no penetration but, I knew where my penis went (or, at least I thought I did). So, I asked Dawn if she was ready to give me a blowjob and she did it. I did not have an orgasm or anything close. I think just the idea of almost getting caught made it fun. Once again, I was famous for getting the first blowjob in class. My friends told everyone and word got around really fast. Now that I think about it, Dawn and I attempted intercourse several times but penetration never happened. For some reason, it never seemed to work. I don't understand why or what happened, it just never seemed to work.

Around this time, my mom brought me a book called Where Did I Come From. I remember the first day when I got the book, we were going on a class trip and my teacher let me read it in the back of the van with the rest of my classmates. I do believe that book was passed around to everyone in the van. It was a pretty nice trip.

When I was reading the book at home, everything seemed to make sense. One of the pages stuck in my head and I can still see the page today. The page has a picture of a man lying on top of a woman with a smile on his face. The caption of the page reads something to the effect of "the closest the man can get to the woman is to put his penis in her vagina.' I must have read that sentence over and over for at least 2 weeks. For some reason, it struck a chord in me and I could never let it go. It was so powerful I can still see the picture in my head today. It had to be around 20 years ago. That's just how powerful it was and still is.

From 6th grade through 9th grade, nothing happened. This had to be my weird stage. I did nothing. I didn't even masturbate or anything. It was like everything just stopped. I just went to school and had fun. My phone would ring and all of that good stuff but all of the touching and stuff pretty much stopped. I used to grab the girl's butts. I do remember that. But, the teachers told the girls to grab out butts back. We still went on the camping trips and all that but nothing happened. I did not have a girlfriend for a few years. I spent many hours playing a role-play video game. It was called Exodus: Ultima 3. (Very cool game at the time!)

I actually had intercourse for the first time in 10th grade. My girlfriend lived down the street and it was our 6-month anniversary. My mom was out for the evening and we broke in our couch. The initial sensation was odd but of course, it felt really good really fast. Then, I felt that pre-ejaculatory sensation in the lower region of my testicles and that was the best. I do remember asking her if it hurt and luckily, there was no blood. I also remember telling her that I would not put it all the way in. Yeah, right! When my orgasm neared, I'm sure I was all the way in. And, just as the stereotype goes, it only lasted for a few minutes.

"Melanie" and I had sex several more times during our relationship. After she started to enjoy herself, she got into it as well. The only one-sided thing was that I would go down on here and she never went down on me. Later, I came to find out she did not want to do it because she did not know how. That's ok. I really can't blame her for that.

Now, this is the funny part. It is because of Melanie that I am now in this field. During our sexual adventures, I noticed she would have orgasms when she was on top and only when she was on top. I wondered why? {That was all it took, believe it or not} Then, the actual event happened that would change my life. It was a rainy Saturday with nothing really to do. I found a book on my mother shelf and I started to read it. It was called Human Sexuality by Masters and Johnson. By Sunday evening, I had finished reading the entire book and many of my questions had been answered. I had also discovered a very important word as well. The word was clitoris. I remembered where it was and I planned to look for it on my girlfriend the next time I was in her area. Well, I was in the process of going down on her and guess what? She had one. I remembered from the book that it was very sensitive and its only job was pleasure. I started to lick it and she started to move around. The next thing I knew she was having an orgasm. She asked me what I did and I told her it was a secret. From that point on, my girlfriend had a constant smile stuck on her face.

Before I left high school, I read a book called How to Conquer the Sensuous Woman. I have no clue who wrote it but I did steal it out of my father desk. I read that book in a few days too. I don't remember what it said to do but it must have been good because I burned through it. I also remember calling a friend about the book but I don't remember his response. I can remember some things but not all.

When I started college, I was really interested in many of the sex books at Barnes and Noble. I bought several of those books. Now, I think I'm up to around 1990 because I went to Penn State. I remember buying Extended Sexual Orgasm (ESO) and The G-Spot. I used to keep them hidden way up high in my closet. For several years, I was really interested in learning about the many opinions that are out there regarding sex and sexuality. I read several books by feminist authors Mary Daly, Gerd Vandenberg and Susan Faludi. (I even read Eve's Rib and Sperm Wars but that was later).

In 1995, when I found out I got accepted to NYU, I went through a Steven King phase. I'm not sure why but it was fun books to read his books. During my time at NYU, did just what my main sexuality professor suggested and I went into the city. I did not get into any of the "hands on" stuff but the exposure was enough. I went to a couple of S&M Clubs (Hellfire Club, The Vault). This professor took my class to a meeting of the Eulenspeigel Society (another S/M group). I ended up buying a pair of latex pants {$210} that I still have.

I was invited to go to the Black and Blue Ball at Roseland. A friend of mine was dancing and she put me on the guest list (very cool). I was dressed as well. I had on my latex pants, leather jacket and boots {I received many compliments on my butt that night}. That was the first time I met B. D. in the flesh. Anyhow, I saw some of the coolest things I have ever seen in my life. There were some people walking around nude, vampires in full dress and some of the most intricate latex gowns on the planet. Some of those gowns cost around $10,000! Really nice stuff. On the other hand, there were people getting spanked, whipped or whatever all over the place. It was intense. Did I partake in the action? No, I just like the atmosphere and the clothes.

I also had an Internet relationship. I met a woman on-line and we started to date. My mom lives in Norfolk VA and she lived in Richmond so she drove down to meet me. We hung around together for the entire day and just had fun. To end the day, she gave me a blowjob that was pretty lame but that was ok. Then, I spent my entire spring break with her. The only thing we did was have sex, see parts of Richmond and have more sex. But the end of my time with her, she was swallowing ejaculate, shaving her Mons bald and she experienced anal intercourse for the first time. With the help of my magic wand, she discovered she could have multiple orgasms. It was fun to watch this sexual being just evolve before your eyes. She never really learned how to give a good blowjob, though. (Well, not with me.)

I guess, now is a good time for me to tell you about my B. D. story. Well, "B" decided to pass on her sexual knowledge to the next generation of educators. A friend from NYU asked me if I would be interested in taking the class. The class cost $300 for 5 weeks and the next thing I knew I was sitting in a circle telling 10 people my masturbation history. That part was fine and I still had my clothes on.

The next week, B began to demonstrate her sex coaching technique on us. She used one woman and one man. She just demonstrated her interviewing technique. That was pretty basic. Nothing to intense for my eyes and I still had my clothes on.

The 3rd week, she demonstrated the genital show and tell. Again, she picked a woman and a guy (I should let you know now that there were only 2 males in the room). My first button was pushed when the woman did the genital show and tell was on her period. That has never been my cup to tea. I did not have a problem with seeing the blood. It was kind of tough for me when she started to masturbate and it was starting to collect near her anus and it was getting all over her fingers. And then, a colleague from NYU asked her to taste and she did. I know when I cut my finger, the first place it goes is in my mouth. So, for a bit, I had to argue with myself regarding the difference between vaginal blood vs. blood from another part of your body.

After that, she demonstrated the genital show and tell on the other guy. At first, I felt kind of funny looking at another man penis for that long. He did not masturbate or anything like that. She got out the mirror and they explored his genitals. No more, no less. We were all sitting in a semi circle and just watching Master B do her thing. She was enjoying herself and I was learning her technique. It was fun. No worries or anything close, until....

Oh wait, I almost forgot about the female ejaculator. B had us practice on each other and I was paired with a woman named "Kathy". Kathy is a pretty big woman; she's taller than I am. So she laid down on the floor and opened her legs. Under closer inspection, I notice a good amount of metal next her Mons. Well, she has her clit pierced not once but a few times. She told me when she is getting fisted, fucked or masturbating, all of the metal starts to vibrate and it gives her a much deeper sensation and pleasure. She said it did not hurt when she got it done. I was impressed.

So, Kathy grabs the magic wand and goes at it. So, I'm just watching and her orgasm nears. When it hits, she tensed up and used her fingers to spread her lips. Out of no place, a clear stream of liquid shot out about a good 4 feet. It was "Cool!" The others saw it and they came over. Surprise, surprise!

She squirted again after a second orgasm but this time, we caught it in a glass. B did not believe it was anything other than urine. We all smelled the glass looking for a urine smell but we could not find anything close. It looked just like water and had no smell what so ever. After a few more orgasms, she ran out but it was still a great experience to say the least.

So, the 4th week started just as all the rest. Just cool, nice and smooth. So, we all sat in the circle and she's asking if we have any questions. The next thing I know, B whips her head around and asks me if I was "ready to go." I was thinking she was going to finish out with the person who she started with last week. She caught me so off guard. 95% of my body was saying no, hell no. It was that 5% that ran up and out of my mouth and said yes. I actually remember asking myself who said yes? I knew my mouth had moved but I don't remember any sound coming out.

Somehow my clothes came off and I was lying on the ground with some friends/colleagues looking at my body. Then, B comes down next to me and she did not have the mirror. From somewhere back in my brain, a message came forward which said 'Hey stupid, you do realize your going to have to masturbate, right?' Boy, oh Boy!

But, B wants to play first. She gets out these rubber vacuum cups and puts them on my nipples to get them up. I was kind of cold so the vacuum cups worked. I got some lube and started to demonstrate my technique. I remember B saying something like "… now, Nick as an interesting technique. See how he kinda twists his wrist on the head." One of the women made a comment like "Ohhh, yes. Interesting." So, I'm just sitting there playing with myself and then, B asks me a question.

"So Nick, have you ever had your prostate stimulated before?" Now, this was when all of buttons were pushed at the same time. I said no and this evil/sinister-type grin came over her face. I knew there was only one way to get to the prostate. She, B gets this dildo (about 3 inches long) and tells the class about anal play and how to play safe. I should also mention I was never able to get an erection either. So, B crawls between my legs and tells me take a deep breath. So, it goes in and I'm still masturbating all the while B seems to be really enjoying herself. Hell, for a second I though she was gonna cum!

I decided to focus on the sensation of the dildo. For years, I had been telling guys about their prostate and how much pleasure could come from it. Well, I now know I am not one of those guys. I was truly searching for an ounce of pleasure but I could find nothing. It was not there. B did ask if I liked it and I told her I wasn't really getting anything out of it. I've accepted the fact that my g-spot does not do anything for me.

After all that, we sat around as a group for a while and just talked. It was a nice way to bring the event to a close. Well, there was one more day of class left. What could happen on the last day of class? My, oh my!

To close this paper, I will have to tell you about the circle jerk. As a group, we called it a 'celebration'. The other guy was not there so I was the only guy in the room. So, here I am sitting in a room full of my nude friends about to so something I usually do in private. Well, B says lets get started and off we went. I was sitting next to the Kathy (the female ejaculator) who was not feeling to well. So, I started to masturbate and a few my friends were sitting across from me, watching me. But again, I did not have an erection. B keeps her place cooler than I would like but it was ok.

Anyhow, I have to say I saw one of the most beautiful vulvas on the planet. She's was a friend of mine from and NYU and her vulva was just amazing. She was masturbating in a circular pattern and I she opened her labia and it was so beautiful. It was a perfect "V" shape with a deep pink color. It was truly eye candy! Lucky for me, she is in one of Betty's videos and I get to see her whenever I choose.

What was really great about the evening was that I was able to enjoy the sounds of pleasure. One woman had around 10 orgasms and she was very vocal. Both of my friends came twice, along with the rest of the women. I just stopped masturbating and just listened to them. I wish I had been able to put it on tape. It was just so amazing. After about an hour, we just sat around and talked and ate fruit.

I have various smaller stories about educating others and being educated by clients but that is all of the major stuff. I hope it was a fun read for you and I'll be seeing you around.

References Section

Chapter 1

Akbar, N. (1979, August) Mental disorder among African-Americans. Paper presented at the 12th Annual National Convention of the Association of Black Psychologists, Atlanta.

Barron, M.L. (1946) People Who Intermarry. Syracuse: Syracuse Univ. Press

Bell, A. (1968) Black Sexuality, fact and fancy. A paper. Black American Series, Indiana University, Bloomington Indiana.

Bernard, J. (1966) Note on educational homogamy in negro-white and white-negro marriages, 1960. Journal of Marriage and the Family, 27, 274-276.

Bowers, W.J. (1974). Executions in America. Lexington Books: New York.

Burt, M. (1983) Cultural myths and supports for rape. Journal of personality and Social Psychology, 38, 217-230.

Chapman, A.B. (1988) Black Families.

Davie, M. (1949) Negroes in American Society. McGraw-Hill: New York, p. 207.

Day, B.P. (1974) Sexual life between Blacks and Whites. Crowell: New York.

Dworkin, A. (1989) Pornography: Men possessing women. Dutton: New York

Epstein, J., Langenbaum, S. (1994) The criminal justice and community response to rape. Washington D.C.: U.S. Department of Justice.

Fanon, F. (1967) Black Skin, White Masks. Grove Press: New York.

Franklin, J.H. (1947) From Slavery to Freedom. Random House: New York.

Frazier, F. E. (1962) Black Bourgeoisie. Crowell-Collier Publishing Co: New York, p. 182.

Gallup, G., Newport, F. (1991) For the first time, more Americans approve of interracial marriages than disapprove. Gallup Monthly Poll, no. 311 Aug., 60-62.

Giacopassi, D.J., Dull, R.T.(1986) Gender and racial differences in the acceptance of rape myths within a college population. Sex Roles, 15, 63-75.

Golden, J. (1959) Facilitating factors in negro-white intermarriage. Social Forces, 36, 273-284.

— (1954) Patterns of negro-white intermarriage. American Sociology Review, 19, 144-147.

— (1953) Characteristics of the negro-white intermarriage in Philadelphia. American Sociology Review, 18, 177-183.

Groth, A. (1979) Men who rape: The psychology of the offender. Plenum Press: New York.

Hernton, C. (1965) Sex and racism in America. Grove Press: New York.

Hirsh, M.D. (1981) Women and violence. Van Nostrand Reinhold: New York.

Hoch, P. (1979). White hero, Black beast: Racism, sexism, and the mask of masculinity. Pluto Press: London.

Hollanson, J.E., Calder, G. (1960) Negro-White Differences on the MMPI. Journal of Chemical Psychology, pp. 32-33.

Hunt, C.L., Collier, R.W. (1957) Intermarriage and cultural change: a study of Philippine_american Marriages. Social Forces, 35, 223-230.

Hursh, C. (1977). The trouble with rape. Nelson-Hall: Chicago.

Lynn, A.Q. (1953) Interracial marriage in Washington D.C., 1940-1947. Ph.D. dissertation Catholic University of America. (unpublished)

Master, W., Johnson, V. (1966) Human Sexual Response. Little, Brown and Co.: Boston

McCaghy, C. (1980) Crime in American society. MacMillian: New York.

McCary, J.L. (1967) Human Sexuality. Van Nostrand: New York.

Merton, R.K. (1941) Intermarriage and the social structure: fact and theory. Psychiatry, 4, 361-374.

Osmundsen, J.A. (1965) Doctor discusses mixed marriage. New York Times, November 7, p.73.

Pavela, T.H. (1964) An exploratory study of negro-white intermarriage in Indiana. Marriage and Family Living, 26, 209-211.

Pettigrew, T. (1964) A Profile of the Negro American. D. Van Nostrand Company: New York, pp. 17-22.

Pierre Van Der Berhe, C.F. (1967) Race and Racism. John Wiley: New York.

Pope, B.R. (1986) Black men in Interracial Relationships: Psychological and Therapeutic Issues. Journal of Multicultural Counseling and Development, 19, 10-16.

Proshansky, H, Newton, P. (1968). Nature and Meaning of Negro—Self-Identification in Social Class, Race and Psychological Development. Holt, Rinehart and Winston: New York.

Risdon, R. (1954) A study of interracial marriages based on data for Los Angeles county. Sociology and Social Research, 39, 92-95.

Schneep, G.J., Yui, A.M. (1955) Cultural and marital adjustment of Japanese war-brides. American Journal of sociology, 61, 48-50.

Schrink, J., LeBeau, J. (1984) Forcible rape: Myths and myth making. Paper presented at the Academy of Criminal Justice Sciences Annual Meeting.

Schwendinger, J., Schwendinger, H. (1968) Rape myths: in legal, theoretical, and everyday practice. Journal of Criminal Law, 59, 559-615.

Staples, R.(1982) Black Masculinity. The Black Scholar Press: San Francisco.

— (1973) The Black Woman in America. Nelson Hall Publishers: Chicago

— (1971) The myth of the impotent black male. The Black Scholar, 2, 2-9.

Surra, C.A. (1991) Research and theory on mate selection and premarital relationships in the 1980's. In Contemporary Families: Looking Forward, Looking Back, ed. A. Booth, 54-75. National Council on Family Relations: Minneapolis.

Varelas, N., Foley, L.A. (1998) Blacks' and Whites' perceptions of Interracial and Interracial date rape. Journal of Social Psychology, 138, 392-400.

Vontress, C. (1971) The Black Male Personality. The Black Scholar, June 1971, 10-16.

Wriggens, J. (1983). Rape, racism, and the law. Harvard Women's Law Journal, 6, 103-141.

Wyatt, G. (1992) The sociocultural context of African American and White American Women's Rape. Journal of Social Issues, 48, 77-91.

Wyatt, G., Strayer, R., Lobitz, W. (1976) Issues in the treatment of sexually dysfunctioning couples of Afro-American descent. Psychotherapy, Theory, Research and Practice, 13, 44-50.

Chapter 2

Bennett, N,B., Bloom, D.E., & Craig, P.H. (1989). The divergence of black and white marriage patterns. *American Journal of Sociology, 95*, pp. 692-722.

Browning, S.L.& Miller, R.R. (1999). Marital messages: The case of black women and their children. *Journal of family Issues, 5*, 633-647.

Bulcroft, R.A., & Bulcroft, K.A. (1993). Race differences in attitudinal and motivational factors in the decision to marry. *Journal of Marriage and Family, 55*, 338-355.

Chadiha, L. (1992). Black husband's economic problems and resiliency during the transition to marriage. *Families in Society, 73,* 542-552.

Cherlin, A.J. (1992). *Marriage, Divorce, Remarriage.* Cambridge, MA: Harvard University Press.

Davis, L.E., & Strube, M.J. (1993). An assessment of romantic commitment among black and white dating couples. *Journal of Applied Social Psychology, 23,* 212-225.

Ellison, R. (1952) *Invisible Man.* New York: Random House.

Franklin, C.W. (1980). White racism as the cause of black male-female conflict: A critique. *Western Journal of Black Studies, 4,* 42-49.

Franklin, C.W. (1989). Black male-female conflict: Individually caused and culturally nurtured. In D.P. Aldridge (ed.). *Black male-female relationships: A resource book of selected materials,* (pp.213-222). Dubuque, IA: Kendall/Hunt.

Frazier, E.F. (1949). *The Negro in the United States.* New York: Macmillan company.

Gary, L. & Leashore, B. (1982). This high risk status of black men. *Social Work, 27,* 54-58.

Guttentag, M., & Second, P. (1983). *Too many women? The sex ratio question,* Beverly Hills, CA: Sage Publications.

Kalmijn, M. (1993). Trends in black/white intermarriage. *Social forces, 72,* 119-146.

Lawrence, G.E. (1986). Predicting interpersonal conflict between men and women, *American Behavioral Scientist, 29,* 635-646.

Majors, R., & Billson, J.M. (1993) *Cool Pose: The dilemmas of black manhood in America.* New York: Simon & Schuster.

Martin, T.C. & Bumpass, L.L. (1989). Recent trends in marital dissolution. *Demography, 26,* 37-51.

Moynihan, P. (1965). *The Negro family: The case for national action.* Washington, DC: U.S. Government Printing Office.

National Institute on Drug Abuse. (1991). *National household survey of drug abuse: highlights 1990 (DHHS Publication No. PDM 91-1732).* Washington, DC: U.S. Government Printing Office.

Rank, M.R. & Davis, L.E. (1996). Perceived happiness outside of marriage among black and white spouses. *Family Relationship, 45,* 435-441.

Rusbult, C., Johnson, D., & Morrow, G. (1986a). Determinants and consequences of exit, voice, loyalty, and neglect: Responses to dissatisfaction in adult romantic involvements. *Human Relations, 39,* 45-63.

Rusbult, C. & Martz, J. (1995). Remaining in an abusive relationship: An investment model analysis of nonvoluntary dependence. *Personality & Social Psychology Bulletin, 21,* 558-571.

Stack, C. (1974). *All our kin: Strategies for survival in a black community.* New York: Harper and Row.

Staples, R. (1978). Masculinity and race: The dual dilemma of Black men. *Journal of Social Issues, 34,* 169-183.

Sweet, J., & Bumpass, L. (1987). *American families and households.* New York: Russell Sage foundation.

Testa, M. & Krogh, M. (1995). The effects of employment on marriage among black males in inner-city Chicago. In B.M. Tucker

& C. Mitchell-Kerman (eds.), *The decline in marriage among African Americans* (pp. 59-95). New York: Russell Sage Foundation.

Thoits, P. (1983). Multiple identities and psychological well-being: A reformation and test of the social isolation hypothesis. *American Sociological Review, 48,* 174-187.

Thomas, V. (1990). Determinants of global life happiness and marital happiness in dual-career black couples. *Family Relations, 39,* 174-178.

Tucker, M.B., & Taylor, R.J. (1996). Gender, age and marital status as related to romantic involvement among African American singles. In J. Jackson & L. Chatters (Eds.), *Family life in black America* (pp. 79-94). Thousand Oaks, CA: Sage Publications.

U.S. Bureau of the Census (1991). *Statistical abstract of the United States.* Washington, DC: U.S. Government Printing Office.

U.S. Bureau of the Census (1994). *Statistical abstract of the United States.* Washington DC: U.S. Government Printing Office.

U.S. Bureau of the Census (1996). *Marital status of persons 15 years old and over by age, sex, region and race: March, 1995. Marital status and living arrangements (current population reports, series P-20).* Washington, DC: U.S. Government Printing Office.

U.S. Department of Justice. (1992). *Correctional populations in the United states, 1990. (Publication No. NCJ-134946).* Washington, DC: U.S. Government Printing Office.

Wilson, W.J. (1987). *The truly disadvantaged: The inner city, the underclass, and public policy.* Chicago: University of Chicago Press.

Wineberg, H. (1994b). *The characteristics of ever-separated black women who attempt a marital reconciliation.* Paper presented at the southern Demographic Association meeting in Atlanta.

Wineberg, H. (1996). The prevalence and characteristics of black having a successful marital reconciliation. *Journal of Divorce & Remarriage, 25,* 75-86.

Chapter 3

Datzman, J. & Gardner, C. (2000). In my mind, we are all humans: Notes on the public management of Black-White interracial romantic relationships. *Marriage and Family Review, 30,* 5-24.

Davis, F. (1991). *Who is Black? One Nation's definition.* The Pennsylvania State University Press.

Kalmijn, M. (1993). Trends in Black/white intermarriage. *Social Forces, 72,* 119-146.

Mathabane, M. & Mathabane, G. (1991). *Love in Black and White: The triumph of love over prejudice.* New York: MacMillian.

Moore, R. (1999). Interracial dating as an indicator of integration. *Black Issues in Higher Education, 15,* 26.

Myrdal, G. (1944). *An American Dilemma: The Negro problem and modern democracy.* Harper-Collins: New York.

Todd, J., McKinney, J., Harris, R., Chadderton, R. & Small, L. (1992). Attitudes toward interracial dating: Effects of age, sex, and race. *Journal of Multicultural Counseling and Development, 20,* 202-208.

Van den Berghe, P. (1967). Hypergamy, Hypergenation and miscegenation. *Human Relations, 13,* 83-91.

Williamson, J. (1980). *New People: Miscegenation and Mulattoes in the United States.* Free Press.

Wirth, L. & Goldhammer, H. (1944). The hybrid and the problem of miscegenation, pp. 253-369, in Klineberg, O. (Ed.) *Characteristics of the American Negro.*

Zebroski, S. (1999). Black-white intermarriages. *Journal of Black Studies, 30,* 123-133.

Chapter 4

"Freshmen survey shows middle of the road trend." June 28, 1986. *Willimantic Chronicle,* P.2.

Greer, W.R. (1986, Nov. 23) Violence against homosexuals rising, groups seeking wider protections. *New York Times,* p.36.

Grossman, A.H. (1991) Gay man and hiv/aids: Understanding the Double Stigma. *JANAC, 2(4),* 28-32.

Herek, G.M. (1984a) Beyond 'homophobia": A social psychological perspective on attitudes toward lesbians and gay men. *Journal of Homosexuality, 10(1/2),* 2-17.

Herek, G.M. (1986) On heterosexual masculinity: Some psychical consequences of the social construction of gender and sexuality. *American Behavioral Scientist, 29,* 563-577.

Herek, G.M., Glunt, E.K. (1993) Interpersonal contact and heterosexuals' attitudes toward gay man: Results from a national survey. *Journal of Sex Research, 30,* 239-244.

Hulbert, J.S. (1989) The southern region: A test of the hypothesis of cultural distinctiveness. *The Sociological Quarterly,* 30, 245-266.

Kinsey, A.C., Pomeroy, W.B., Martin, C.E., Gebhard, P.H. (1948). *Sexual behavior in the human male.* Philadelphia: Saunders.

Kite, M.E. (1984) Sex differences in attitudes toward homosexuals: A meta-analysis review. *Journal of Homosexuality, 3,* 107-121.

Marsiglio, W. (1993) Attitudes toward homosexual activity and gays as friends: A national survey of heterosexual 15 to 19 year old males. *Journal of Sex Research, 30,* 12-17.

National Gay Task Force. (1984) *Anti-gay/lesbian victimization.* Washington, DC: Author. (Available from National Gay Task Force, 1517 U Street, NW, Washington, DC 20009)

National Gay Task Force (1988) *Anti-gay/lesbian victimization, and defamation in 1987.* Washington DC: Author. (Available from National Gay Task Force, 1517 U Street, NW, Washington, DC 20009)

Page,S., Yee, M. (1986) Conception of male and female homosexual stereotypes among university undergraduates. *Journal of Homosexuality, 12,* 109-118.

"Public perceptions of gays: Few changes in the past 5 years." Dec. 6, 1982. *Sexuality Today,* p.1.

Richmond-Abbot, M. (1992). *Masculine & feminine: Gender roles over the life cycle.* 2nd ed. New York: McGraw-Hill

Rushing, W. (1979). The functional importance of sex roles and sex related behavior in societal reactions to residual deviance. *Journal of Health and Social Behavior, 20,* 208-217.

St. Lawrence, J., Husfeld, B., Kelly, J., Hood, H., Smith, S. (1990). The stigma of aids: Fear of disease and prejudice toward gay men. *Journal of Homosexuality, 19(3),* 85-101.

Staff. (1990, Winter). Some facts on suicide and gay youth. *Momentum*, p.1

Wells, J.W., Kline, W.B. (1987). Self—disclosure of homosexual orientation. *Journal of Social Psychology, 127*, 191-197.

Chapter 5

Anderson, J.D., (1994) School climate for gay and lesbian students and staff members. *Phi Delta Kappan, 76(2)*, 151-154.

Anderson, S., Henderson, D. (1985) Working with lesbian alcoholics. Social Work, 30(6), 518-524.

Bell, A., Weinberg, M.S. (1978) *Homosexualities: A study of diversity among men and women.* New York: Simon and Schuster.

Burke, P. (1982) *Bar use and alienation in lesbians and heterosexual women alcoholics.* Paper presented at the Thirteith National Alcoholism Forum, Washington, DC.

Chafetz, J.S. (1974) "A study of homosexual women". *Social Work, 19(6)*, 714-723.

Comstock, G.D. (1989) Victims of anti-gay/lesbian violence. *Journal of Interpersonal Violence, 4*, 101-106.

D'Augelli, A.R. (1992) Lesbian and gay male undergraduates' experience of harassment and fear on campus. *Journal of Interpersonal Violence, 7*, 383-395.

Dressler, J. (1985) Survey of school preicipals regarding alleged homosexual teachers in the classroom: How likely (really) is discharge?. *University of Dayton LawReview, 10(3)*, 599-620.

Eberle, P.H. (1982) Alcohol abusers and non-users: A discriminant analysis of differences between two subgroups of batterers. *Journal of Health and Social Behavior, 23*, 260-271.

Fifield, L. (1980) *Alcoholism and the gay community.* Paper presented at the meeting of the National Coalition of Alcoholism, Seattle, WA.

Frieze, I., & Knoble, J. (1980) *The effects of alcohol on marital violence.* Presented at the Annual Meeting of the American Psychological Association. Montreal, P.Q., Canada, September.

Gallup, G. (1977) *"But make exception in case of certain jobs: Majority support equal rights in principal of hiring homosexuals."* Chicago: Field Newspaper Syndicate.

Goffman, E. (1963) *Stigma: Notes on the management of spoiled identity.* Englewood Cliffs, N.J.: Prentice-Hall.

Grosselin, R., Nice, S. (1987) *Lesbian and gay issues in early recovery.* Center City: Hazelden.

Hunter, J., & Schaecher, R. (1990) Lesbian and gay youth. In M.J. Rotheram-Borus, *Planning to live: Evaluating and treating suicidal teens in community settings.* (pp. 297-316). Tulsa: University of Oklahoma Press.

Israelstam, S. & Lambert, S. (1984) Gay Bars. *Journal of Drug Issues, 14*, 637-653.

Khayatt, D. (1990) Legalized Invisibility: The effect of Bill 7 on lesbian teachers. *Women's Studies International Forum, 13(3)*, 185-193.

Kus, R.J. (1990) *Keys to caring: Assisting your gay and lesbian clients.* Boston: Alyson, Publications, Inc.

Levine, M.P., Leonard, R. (1984) Discrimination against lesbians in the work force. *Journal of Women in Culture and Society*, *9(4)*, 700-710.

Levitt, E.E., Klassen, A.D. (1974) Public attitude toward homosexuality. *Journal of Homosexuality*, *1*, 29-43.

Levitt, E.E., Klassen, A.D. (1974) "Public attitudes towards homosexuals: Part of the 1970 national survey of the Institute for Sex Research." *Journal of Homosexuality*,*1*,131-139.

Lockhart, L.L., White, B.W., Causby, V., Issac, A. (1994) Letting out the secret: Violence in lesbian relationships. *Journal of Interpersonal Violence*, *9(4)*, 469-492.

New York City Gay and Lesbian Anti-Violence Project (1995) *Stop the violence*, *6(1)*, Winter/Spring.

Nardi, P.M. (1982) Alcoholism and homosexuality: A theoretical perspective. *Journal of Homosexuality*, *7*, 9-25.

Olson, M.R. (1987) A study of gay and lesbian teachers. *Journal of Homosexuality*, *13(4)*, 73-81.

Rosario, M., Rotheram-Borus, M.J., Reid, H. (1992) *Personal resources, gay-related stress, and multiple problems behaviors among gay and bisexual male adolescents*. Unpublished manuscript, Columbia University.

Saghir, M.T., Robins, E. (1973) *Male and female homosexuality*. Baltimore: The William L. Wilkens Company.

Schilit, R., Lie, G., Montagne, M. (1990) Substance use as a correlate of violence in intimate lesbian relationships. *Journal of Homosexuality*, *19(3)*, 51-65.

Zoglin, R. (1974) *"The Homosexual Executive."* MBA (July-August): 26-31.

Chapter 6

Allen, L. & Gorski, R. (1992). Sexual orientation and the size of the anterior commissure in the human brain. *Proceedings of the National Academy of Science, 89,* 7199-7202.

Bailey, J.M. (1996). Gender identity. In R.C. Savin-Williams & K.M. Cohen (Eds.), *The lives of lesbians, gays, and bisexuals: Children to adults* (pp.71-93).

Bailey, J.M., Bobrow, D., Wolfe, M. & Mikach, S. (1995). Sexual orientation of adult sons of gay father. *Developmental Psychology, 31,* 124-129.

Bailey, J.M. & Pillard, R.C. (1991). A genetic study of male sexual orientation. *Archives of General Psychiatry, 48,* 1089-1096.

Bailey, J.M. & Zucker, K.J. (1995). Childhood sex-typed behavior and sexual orientation: A conceptual analysis and quantitative review. *Developmental Psychology, 31,* 43-55.

Beach, F. (1950). Comments on the second dialogue in Corydon. In Gide, A., Corydon, Farrar, Straus: New York.

Baldwin, J.D. & Baldwin, J.J. (1997). Gender differences in sexual interest. *Archives of Sexual Behavior, 26,* 181-210.

Bell, A.P. & Weinberg, M.S. (1978). *Homosexualiities: A study of diversity among men and women.* New York: Simon & Schuster.

Bell, A.P. & Weinberg, M.S. & Hammersmith, S.K. (1981). *Sexual Preference.* Indiana University Press: Bloomington, IN.

Bem, S. L. (1981). *Bem sex-role inventory' professional manual.* Consulting Psychologists Press: Palo Alto, CA.

Berger, P. & Luckmann, T. (1966). *The social construction of reality: A treatise in the sociology of knowledge.* Doubleday: Garden City, NY.

Berkey, B.R., Perelman-Hall, T., & Kurdek, L.A. (1990). The multidimensional scale of sexuality. *Journal of Homosexuality*, 19, 67-87.

Bieber, I. (1962). *Homosexuality.* Basic Books: New York, NY.

Blackwood, E. (1993). Breaking the mirror: The construction of lesbianism and the antorpological discourse on homosexuality. In D.N. Suggs & A.W. Miracle (Eds.) *Culture and Human Sexuality* (pp.328-340).

Blumstein, P.W. & Schwartz, P. (1976). Bisexuality in men. *Urban Life*, 5, 339-358.

Blumstein, P.W. & Schwartz, P. (1990). Intimate relationships and the creation of sexuality. In D.P. McWhirter, S.A. Sanders & J. M. Reinisch (Eds.) *Homosexuality/Heterosexuality: Concepts of sexual orientation* (pp. 307-320). Oxford University Press: New York.

Boxer, A. & Cohler, B. (1989). The life course of gay and lesbian youth: An immodest proposal for the study of lives. *Journal of Homosexuality*, 17, 315-355.

Brown, Lesbian I dentities: Conceptual issues. In A.R. 'Aggelli & C.J. Pattersons (Eds.) *Lesbian, gay and bisexual identities across the lifespan: Psychological perspectives.* Oxford University Press: New York.

Bullough, V. (1990). The Kinsey Scale in historical perspective. In McWhirter, D.P., Saunders, S.A.and Reinich, J.M. (eds.), Homosexuality/*Heterosexuality: Concepts of Sexual Orientation*. Oxford University Press: New York.

Carpenter, E. (1894). *Homogenic Love and Its Place in a Free Society*, Labour Press, Manchester, England.

Cass, V.C. (1979). Homosexual identity formation: A theoretical model. *Journal of Homosexuality*, 4, 219-235.

Cass, V.C. (1983). Homosexual identity: A concept in need of defense. *Journal of Homosexuality*, 11, 105-126.

Cass, V.C. (1990). The implication of homosexual identity formation for the Kinsey model and the scale of sexual preference. In McWhirter, D.P., Saunders, S.A.and Reinich, J.M. (eds.), *Homosexuality/Heterosexuality: Concepts of Sexual Orientation*. Oxford University Press: New York.

Cass, V.C. (1996). Sexual orientation identity formation: A western phenomenon. In R.P. Cabaj & T.S. Stein (Eds.) *Textbook of Homosexuality and Mental Health* (pp.227-251).

Chapman, B.E. & Brannock, J.C. (1987). Proposed model of lesbian identity development: An empirical examination. *Journal of Homosexuality*, 14, 69-80.

Chung, Y. & Katayama, M. (1996). Assessment of sexual orientation in Lesbian/Gay/Bisexual studies. *Journal of Homosexuality*, 30, 1996.

Coleman, E. (1987). Assessment of sexual orientation. Journal of Homosexuality, 14, 9-24.

Committee on Lesbian and Gay Concerns (1991). Avoiding heterosexual bias in language. *American Psychologists*, 46, 973-974.

D'Augelli, A. R. (1989). Lesbians' and gay men's experiences of discrimination and harassment and fear on campus. *Journal of Interpersonal Violence*, 7, 383-395.

DeLamater, J. & Shibley-Hyde, J. (1998). Essentialism vs. sSocial Constructionism in the study of human sexuality. *Journal of Sex Research*, 35, 10-18.

Diamond, M. (1993). Homosexuality and Bisexuality in Different Populations. *Archives of Sexual Behavior*, 22, 291-310.

Diamond, L.M. (2000). Sexual identities, attractions, and behavior among sexual-minority women over a two-year period. *Developmental Psychology*, 36, 241-250.

Diamond, M & Savin-Williams, R.C. (2000). Explaining diversity in the development of same-sex sexuality among young women. *Journal of Social Issues*, 56, 297-313.

Dorner. G. (1975). A neuroendocrine predisposition for homosexuality in men. *Archives of Sexual Behavior*, 4, 1-8.

Dorner, G., Poppe, I., Stahl, F. Kolzsch, J. & Uebelhack, R. (1991). Gene-and environment-dependent neuroendocrine etiogenesis of homosexuality and transsexualism. *Experimental and Clinical Endocrinology*, 98, 141-150.

Ellis, H. & Symonds, J.A. (1896). *Sexual Inversion*, Wilson and Mac-Millian, London.

Fausto-Sterling, A. (1986). *Myths of gender*. Basic Books: New York, NY.

Gagnon, J.H. (1990). The explicit and implicit use of the scripting perspective in sex research. *Annual Review of Sex Research*, 1, 1-43.

Glaude, B.A. (1984). Neuroendocrine response to estrogen and sexual orientation. *Science*, 225, 1496-1498.

Glaude, B.A. & Bailey, J.M. (1995). Spatial ability, handedness, and human sexual orientation. *Psychoneuroendocrinology*, 20, 487-497.

Golden, C. (1987). Diversity and variability in women's sexual identity. In The Boston Lesbian Psychologies Collective (Eds.), *Lesbian psychologies: explorations and challenges* (pp.18-34). Urbana, IL: University of Illinois Press.

Green, R. (1987). *The "sissy boy syndrome" and the development of homosexuality.* Yale University Press: New Haven, CT.

Garnets, L.D. & Peplau, L.A. (2000). Understanding women's sexualities and sexual orientations. *Journal of Social Issues*, 56, 181-192.

Halpin, S. & Allen, M. (2004). Changes in psychosocial well-being during stages of gay identity development. *Journal of Homosexuality*, 47, 109-126.

Hamer, D.H., Hu, S., Magnuson, V.L., Hu, N. & Pattatucci, A. (1993). A linkage between DNA markers on the X chromosome and male sexual orientation. *Science*, 261, 321-327.

Hatterer, L. (1970). *Changing homosexuality in the male.* McGraw-Hill: New York.

Herdt, G. (1984). *Ritualized homosexuality in Melanesia.* University of California Press: Berkeley, CA.

Irvine, J.M. (1990). *Disorders of desire: Sex and gender in modern American sexology.* Temple University Press: Philadelphia, PA.

Katz, N. (1992). *Gay American history: Lesbians and Gay men in the United States.* Meridian: New York.

Kinsey, A., Pomerpy, W., & Martin, C. (1948). *Sexual behavior in the human male.* Philadelphia: W.B. Saunders.

Kinsey, A., Pomerpy, W., & Martin, C. (1948). *Sexual behavior in the human female.* Philadelphia: W.B. Saunders.

Kitzinger, C. & Wilkinson, S. (1995). Transitions from heterosexuality to lesbianism: The discursive production of lesbian identities. *Development Psychology*, 31, 95-104.

Klein, F. Sepekoff, B. & Wolf, T.J. (1985). Sexual orientation: A multi-variable dynamic process. *Journal of Homosexuality*, 11, 35-49.

Kolodny, R.C., Masters, W.H., Hendryx, J. & Toro, G. (1971). Plasma testosterone and semen analysis in male homosexuals. *New England Journal of Medicine*, 285, 1170-1174.

Kolodny, R.C., Jacobs, L.S. Masters, W.H., Toro, G. & Daughaday, W.H. (1972). Plasma gonadotrophins and prolactic in male homosexuals. *Lancet*, 2, 18-20.

Kraft-Ebing, R.V. (1886). *Psychopathia Sexualis: Eine klinisch-Forensische studie*, Enke, Stuttgart, Germany.

Lee, R.M. (1993). *Doing research on sensitive topics.* Sage: London.

LeVey, S. (1991). A difference in hypothalamic structures between heterosexual and homosexual men. *Science*, 253, 1034-1037.

LeVay, S. (1993). *The Sexual Brain.* MIT Press: Cambridge, MA.

Marmor, J. Homosexuality: Is etiology really important. *Journal of Gay and Lesbian Psychotherapy*, 2, 19-28.

Masters, W. H. & Johnson, V.E. (1979). *Homosexuality in Perspective.* Little& Brown: Boston,

Mayne, X. (1908). *The Intersexes: A History of similsexualism as a Problem in Social Life.* Privately printed, Paris.

Mayr, E. (1982). *The growth of biological thought: Diversity, evolution, and inheritance.* Harvard University Press: Cambridge, MA.

McDonald, G.J. (1982). Individual differences in the coming out process for gay men: Implication for theoretical models. *Journal of Homosexuality*, 8, 47-60.

Meyer-Bahlburg, H., Ehrhardt, A. Rosen, L. & Gruen, R. (1995). Prenatal estrogens and the development of homosexual orientatin. *Developmental Psychology*, 31, 17-21.

Minton, H.L. & McDonald, G.J. (1984). Homosexual identity formation as a development process. *Journal of Homosexuality*, 9, 91-104.

National Institutes of Mental Health (1987). *National lesbian health cares survey.* Washington, DC: U.S. Department of Health and Human Services.

Peplau, L.A. & Garnets, L.D. (2000). A new paradigm for understanding women's sexuality and sexual orientation. *Journal of Social Issues*, 56, 329-350.

Philips. G. & Over, R. (1992). Adult sexual orientation in relation to memories of childhood gender conforming and gender nonconforming behaviors. *Archives of Sexual Behavior*, 21, 543-558.

Philips, G. & Over, R. (1995). Differences between heterosexual, bisexual, and lesbian women in recalled childhood experiences. *Archives of Sexual Behavior*, 24, 1-20.

Pillard, R.C., Rosen, L., Meyer-Bahlburgm H., Weinrish, J., Feldman, J. Gruen, R. & ehrhardt, A. (1993). Psychopathology and social functioning in men prenatally exposed to diethylstilbestrol (DES). *Psychosomatic Medicine*, 55, 485-491.

Ponse, B. (1978). *Identities in the lesbian world: The social construction of self.* Greenwood Press: Westport, CT.

Regan, P.C. & Berscheid, E. (1996). Beliefs about the state, goals, and objects of sexual desire. *Journal of Sex and Marital Therapy*, 22, 110-120.

Reynolds, A. & Hanjorgiris, W.F. (2000). Coming out: Lesbian, and gay and bisexual identity development. In R.M. Perez, K.A. DeBord & K.J. Bieschke (Eds.), *Handbook of counseling and psychotherapy with lesbian, gay and bisexual clients* (pp.35-56). American Psychological Association: Washington, DC.

Robinson, V. (1936). *Encyclopedia Sexualis*. Dingwall-Rock: New York, NY.

Rust, P. (1996). Finding a sexual identity and community: Therapeutic implications and cu,tural assumptions in scientific models of coming out. In E.D. Rothblum & L.A. Bond (Eds.), *Preventing heterosexism and homophobia* (pp.87-123). Sage: Thousand Oaks, CA.

Rust, P. (1992). The politics of sexual identity: Sex attraction and behavior formation among lesbians and bisexual women. *Social Problems*, 39, 366-386.

Savin-Williams, R.C. (1990). *Gay and lesbian youth: Expressions of identity.* Hemisphere: Washington DC.

Savin-Williams, R.C. (1994). Verbal and physical abuse as stressors in the lives of lesbian, gay male, and bisexual youths: Associations with school problems, running away, substance abuse, prostitution, and suicide. *Journal of Consulting and Clinical Psychology*, 62, 261-269.

Savin-Williams, R.C. (1995). An exploratory study of pubertal maturation timing and self-esteem among and gay and bisexual male youths. *Developmental Psychology*, 31, 56-64.

Sell, R.L. (1997). Defining and Measuring Sexual Orientation: A Review. *Archives of Sexual Behavior*, 26, 643-658.

Sell, R.L. & Petrulio, C. (1995). Sampling homosexual, bisexual, gays and lesbians for public health research: A review of the literature from 1990-1992. *Journal of Homosexuality*, 30, 31-47.

Shively, M.G., Jones, C., & DeCecco, J.P. (1984). Research on sexual orientation: Definitions and methods. *Journal of Homosexuality*, 9, 29-39.

Shively, M.G. & DeCecco, J.P. (1977). Components of sexual identity. *Journal of Homosexuality*, 3, 41-48.

Siegelman, M. (1974). Parental background of male homosexuals and heterosexuals. *Archives of Sexual Behavior*, 3, 3-38.

Simon, W. & Gagnon, J. H. (1973). *Sexual Conduct*. Aldine: Chicago, Ill.

Silverstein, C. (1977). Homosexuality and the ethics of behavioral intervention: Paper 2. *Journal of Homosexuality*, 2, 205-211.

Smith, E.M., Johnson, S.R., & Guenther, S.M. (1985). Health care attitudes and experiences during gynecologic care among lesbians and bisexuals. *American Journal of Public Health*, 75, 1085-1087.

Socarides, C. (1968*). The Overt Homosexual.* Grune & Stratton: New York, NY.

Sophie, J. (1986). A critical examination of stage theories of lesbian identity development. *Journal of Homosexuality,* 12, 39-51.

Storms, M.D. (1978). Sexual orientation and self-perception. In P. Plinger, K.R. Blanstein, I.M. Spigel, T. Alloway & L. Krames (Eds.) *Advances in the study of communication and affect: Vol. 5. Perception of emotion in self and others.* Plenum: New York.

Storms, M.D. (1980). Theories of sexual orientation. *Journal of Personal Social Psychology,* 38, 783-792.

Swaab, D. & Hofman, M. (1990). An enlarged suprachiasmatic nucleus in homosexual men. *Brain Research,* 537, 141-148.

Tentler, T.N. (1977). *Sin and confession on the eve of the Reformation.* Princeton University Press: Princeton, NJ.

Thompson, N.L., Schwartz, D.M., McCandless, B.R & Edwards, D. (1973). Parent-child relationships and sexual identity in male and female homosexuals and heterosexuals. *Journal of Consulting and Clinical Psychology,* 41, 120-127.

Troiden, R.R. (1979). Becoming homosexual: A model of gay identity acquisition. *Psychiatry,* 42, 362-373.

Ulrichs, K.H. (1994*). The Riddle of Man-Manly Love.* Prometheus Books, Buffalo, NY.

Weinberg, M.S. (1994). Homosexual samples: Differences and similarities. *Journal of Sex Research,* 6, 312-325.

Weinrich, J.D. (1994). Homosexuality. In Bullough, V.L. and Bullough, B. (eds.), *Human Sexuality: An Encyclopedia.* Garland: New York,NY.

Whitam, F.L., Diamond, M. & Martin, J. (1993). Homosexual orientation in twins: A report of 61 pairs and three triples sets. *Archives of Sexual Behavior*, 22, 187-206.

Chapter 7

Ajzen, I. & Fishbein, M. (1975). *Belief, Attitude, Intention and behavior: An introduction to theory and research*. Mass: Addison-Wesley.

Ajzen, I. & Fishbein, M. (1980). *Understanding attitudes and predicting social behavior*. New Jersey: Prentice Hall.

Baker, S., Morrison, D., Carter, W. & Verdon, M. (1996). Using the Theory of Reasoned Action to understand the decision to use condoms in an STD clinic population. *Health Education Quarterly*, 23(4), 528-542.

Baldwin, J.D. & Baldwin, J. I... (1988). Factors affecting AIDS-related sexual risk-taking behavior among college students. *The Journal of Sex Research*, 25, 185-196.

Bandura, A. (1986). Self-efficacy mechanism in physiological activation and health-promoting behavior, in Madden, I., Matthysse, S., Barchas, J. (eds); *Adaptation, Learning and Affect*. New York: Raven Press.

Basen-Engquist, K. & Parcel, G. (1992). Attitudes, Norms, and Self-Efficacy: A model of Adolescents' HIV-related sexual risk behavior. *Health Education Quarterly*, 19(2), 263-277.

Baum, A. & Nesselhof, S.E. (1988). Psychological research and prevention, etiology and treatment of AIDS. *American Psychologist*, 43, 900-906.

Bentler, P.M. & Speckart, G. (1986). Models of attitude-behavior relations. *Psychology Review*, 86, 452-464.

Bogart, L., Cecil, H. & Pinkerton, S. (2000). *Journal of Applied Social Psychology, 30*, 1923-1953.

Bryan, A., Aiken, L. & West, S. (1996). Increasing condom use: Evaluation of a theory-based intervention to prevent sexually transmitted diseases in young women. *Health Psychology, 15*, 371-382.

Calamidas, E.G. (1990). AIDS and STD education: What's really happening in our schools? *Journal of Sex Education and Therapy, 16*, 54-63.

Catania, J.A., Coates, T.J. Kegeles, S. Fullilove, M.T. Peterson, J., Siegel, D. & Hulley, S. (1992). Condom use in multi-ethnic neighborhoods of Dan Francisco: The population-based AMEN (AIDS inn Multi-Ethnic Neighborhoods) Study. *American Journal of Public Health, 82*, 284-287.

Centers for Disease Control (1994, June). *HIV/AIDS surveillance report.* Atlanta, GA: center for Infectious Diseases, Center for Disease Control and Prevention.

Coates, T.J. (1990). Strategies for modifying sexual behavior for primary and secondary prevention of HIV disease. *Journal of Consulting and Clinical Psychology, 58*, 57-69.

Crawford, T.J. & Boyer, R. (1985). Salient consequences, cultural values and childbearing intentions. *Journal of Applied Social Psychology, 15*, 16-30.

Davidson, A. R. & Morrison, D.M. (1983). Predicting contraceptive behavior from attitudes: A comparison of within-versus across-subjects procedures. *Journal of Personality and Social Psychology, 45*, 997-1009.

Emmons, C.A., Joseph, J.G., Kessler, R.C., Wortman, C.B., Montgomery, S.B. & Ostrow, D.G. (1986). Psychosocial predictors of reported behavior change in homosexual men at risk for AIDS. *Health Education Quarterly, 13*, 331-345.

Fisher, J. & Fisher, W. (1992). Changing AIDS risk behavior. *Psychological Bulletin, 111*, 455-474.

Fisher, W., Fisher, J. & Rye, B. (1995). Understanding and promoting AIDS-Preventive behavior: Insights from the theory of Reasoned Action. *Health Psychology, 14*, 225-264.

Holroyd, K., Penzien, D. & Hursey, D. (1984). Change mechanisms in EMG biofeedback training: Cognitive changes underlying improvement in tension headache. *Journal of Consulting Clinical Psychology, 52*, 1039-1053

Kelly, J.A., St. Lawrence, J.S., Brasfield, T.L., Stevenson, L.Y., Diaz, Y.Y. & Hauth, A.C. (1990). AIDS risk behavior patterns among gay men in small southern cities. *American Journal of Public Health, 80(4)*, 416-418.

Kelly, J. St. Lawrence, J., Diaz, Y., Stevenson, L., Hauth, A., Brasfield, T., Kalichman, S., Smith, J. & Andrew, M. (1991). HIV risk behavior reduction following intervention with key opinion leaders of population: An experimental analysis. *American Journal of Public Health, 81*, 168-171.

Moore, S.M. & Rosenthal, D.A. (1991). Adolescents' perception of friends' and parents' attitudes to sex and sexual risk-taking. *Journal of Community and Applied Social Psychology, 1*, 189-200.

O'Keeffe, M., Nasselhof-Kendall, S. & Baum, A. (1990). Behavior and prevention of AIDS: Bases of research and intervention. *Personality and Social Psychology Bulletin, 16*, 166-180.

Perry, M., Sikkema, K. Wagstaff, D., Crumble, D., Solomon, L. Norman, A., Cargill, V., Anderson, E., Kelly, J., Roffman, R., Mercer, M., Winett, R. & Heckman, T. (1996). *Perception and use of the female condom among inner-city woman.* Poster presented at the International Conference on AIDS, Vancouver, Canada.

Shulkin, J., Mayer, J., Wessel, L., de Moor, C., Elder, J. & Franzini, L. (1991). Effects of peer-led AIDS intervention with university students. *Journal of American College Health, 40*, 75-79.

Smetana, J.G. & Adler, N.E. (1980). Fishbein's value x expectancy model: An examination of some assumptions. *Personality Social Psychology Bulletin, 6*, 89-96.

Turtle, A.M., Ford, B., Habgood, R., Grant, M., Bekiaris, J., Constantinou, C., Macek, M. & Polyzoids, H. (1989). AIDS-related beliefs and behaviors of Australian university students. *Medical Journal of Australia, 150*, 371-376.

Walter, H.J., Vaughan, R.D., Gladis, M.M. & Ragin, D.F. (1993). Factors associated with AIDS-related behaviors intentions among high school students in an AIDS epicenter. *Health Education Quarterly, 20*, 409-420.

Winslow, R., Franzini, L. & Hwang, J. (1992). Perceived peer norms, casual sex, and AIDS risk prevention. *Journal of Applied Social Psychology, 22*, 1809-1827.

Wulfert, E. & Wan, C.K. (1993). Condom use: A self-efficacy model. *Health Psychology, 12*, 346-353.

Chapter 8

Altman, L.K. (1991, June 18). W.H.O. says 40 million will be infected with AIDS. *The New York Times*, p B8.

Bennett, W.J. (1988). Sex and the education of our children. *Curriculum review, 27*, 70-130.

Blinn-Pike, L. (1999). Why abstinent adolescents report they have not had sex: understanding sexually resilient youth. *Family Relations, 48*, 295-301.

Brindis, C. (1990). Helping teens wait: abstinence education. *Family Life Educator, 9*, 11-25.

Butterfield, F. (1992, February). U.S. expands its lead in the rate of imprisonment. *The New York Times*, p. C18.

Centers for Disease Control and Prevention (1996). *HIV/AIDS Surveillance Report*. Rockville, MD, U.S. Department of Health and Human Services.

Centers for Disease Control and Prevention (1997). *Division of STD Prevention: Sexually Transmitted Disease Surveillance 1996*. Atlanta, U.S. department of Health and Human Services.

Clowes, B. (1994). *The Pro-Life Activist's Encyclopedia*. Stafford, VA, American Life League.

Denny, G., Young, M., spear, C. (1999) An evaluation of the Sex Can Wait abstinence education curriculum series. *American Journal of Health Behavior, 23*, 134-143.

Gahr, E. (1992). Opposing conceptions of condoms in the schools. *Insights*, Oct., 10-13, 34-36.

Griffin, G.C. (1993). Condom and contraceptives in junior high and high school clinics: What do you think? *Postgraduate Medicine, 93*, 21-38.

Howard, M., McCabe, J.B. (1990). Helping teenagers postpone sexual involvement. *Family Planning Perspectives, 22,* 21-26.

Kelly, M. (1988) *Teens and Chastity: A talk with Molly Kelly* (public school version). Videotape. New Jersey, Monitor Communications.

Khouzam, H.R. (1995). Promotion of sexual abstinence: Reducing adolescent sexual activity and pregnancy. *South Medical Journal, 88*, 709-711.

Kirby, D., Korpi, M., Barth, R.P., & Cagampang, H.H. (1997). The impact of postponing sexual involvement curriculum among youths in California. *Family Planning Perspectives, 29*, 100-108.

Kirby, D. & Scales, P. (1981). An analysis of state guidelines for sex education instruction in public schools. *Family Relations, 30*, 229-237.

Koop, C.E. (1988). AIDS and teenagers: Emerging issues. (Hearing before the select Committee on Children, Youth, and Families: House of Representatives, One-Hundredth Congress, First Session). Washington, DC: Superintendent of Documents, U.S. Government Printing Office.

Lowry, D.T. & Towels, D.E. (1989a). Soap opera portrayals of sex, contraception, and sexually transmitted diseases. *Journal of Communication, 39*, 76-83.

Lowry, D.T. & Towels, D.E. (1989b). Prime time TV portrayals of sex, contraception and venereal disease. *Journalism Quarterly, 66*, 347-352.

Mindus, D. (2000, September 11) What to tell the children: The battle of sex ed. *National Review*, 44-46.

Morse, J. (1999, October 18). Preaching chastity in the classroom. *Time*, 78-80.

New York State Catholic Bishops (1993). New York State Catholic bishops explain why they oppose distribution of condoms to high school students. *The Tablet*, January 30, 12-13.

Olsen, T., Wallace, C. & Miller, B. (1984). Primary prevention of adolescent pregnancy: Promoting family involvement through a school curriculum. *Journal of Primary Prevention, 5*, 75-91.

Olsen, J., Weed, S., Nielsen, A., & Jensen, L. (1992). Student evaluation of sex education programs advocating abstinence. *Adolescence, 27*, 369-380.

Ornstein, A.C. & Levine, D.U. (1993). *Foundations of Education* (5th ed.). Boston, MA: Houghton Mifflin.

Perry, C.L., Kelder, S.H., & Komro, K.A. (1993). The social world of adolescence: family, peers, schools and community. In S. Millstein, A Petersen & E. Nightingale (Eds.) *Promoting the health of adolescence: New directions for the 21st century*. Pp.73-97. New York: Oxford.

SIECUS (1992). SIECUS Fact sheet #3 on comprehensive sexuality education: Sexuality education and the school-issues and answers. *SIECUS Report, 20*.

Ventura, S.J., Martin, J.A., Mathews, T.J., & Clarke, S.C. (1996). Advance report of final natality statistics. *Monthly Vital Statistics Report, 44* (Suppl. 11), S3-S5. Hyattsville, MS: National Center for Health statistics.

Young, M., Core-Gebhart, P., Marx, D. (1992) Abstinence-oriented sexually education: Initial field test results of the Living smart curriculum. *Family Life Educator, 10*, 4-8.

Chapter 9

Abarbanel, A. R. (1978). Diagnoses and treatment of coital discomfort. In J. LoPiccolo & L. LoPiccolo (Eds), *Handbook of Sex Therapy*. New York: Plenum.

American Psychiatric Association. (1987) *Diagnostic and statistical manual of mental disorders*. 3rd edition. Washington, D.C.: American Psychiatric Association.

Anderson, B.L. & Cyranowski, J.M. (1995). Women's sexuality behaviors, responses, and individual differences. *Journal of Consulting Clinical Psychology, 63*, 891-906.

Ashman, R.B. & Ott, A.K. (1989). Auto-immunity as a factor in recurrent vaginal candidosis and the minor vestibular gland syndrome. *Journal of Reproductive Medicine, 34*, 264-266.

Bachman, G., Leiblum, S., Kenmmann, E., Colburn, D. Schwartzman, L. & Shelden, R. (1984). Vaginal atrophy in post-menopausal dyspareunia. *Female Patient, 9*, 118-127.

Bancroft J. & Coles, I. (1976). Three years' experience in a sexual problems clinic. *British Medical Journal, 1,* 1575-1577.

Beard, R.W., Reginald, P.W. & Wadsworth, J. (1988). Clinical features of women with chronic lower abdominal pain and pelvic congestion. *British Journal of Obstetrician and Gynecology, 95,* 152-161.

Ellery, R.S. (1954). Frigidity and dyspareunia. Medical Journal of Austin, 2, 626-628.

Butcher, J. (1999). ABC of sexual health: Female sexual problems II: Sexual pain. *British Medical Journal, 18, 3,* 110-112.

Caird, W. (1988). Modification of urinary urgency. *The Journal of Sex Research, 24,* 183-187.

Chaiken, D., Blaivas, J. & Blaivas, S. (1993). Behavioral therapy for the treatment of refractory interstitial cystitis. *Journal of Urology, 149,* 1445-1448.

Crenshaw, T.L. & Kessler, J. (1985). Vaginismus. *Medical Aspects of Human Sexuality, 19,* 21-32.

Dewitt, D.E. (1991). Dypareunia: Tracing the cause. *Post-Graduate Medicine, 89,* 8, 70, 73.

Fink, P.J. (1972). Dyspareunia: Current concepts. *Medical Aspects of Human Sexuality, 8,* 28-45.

Fitzpatrick, C. DeLancey, J., Elkins, T & McGuire, E. (1993). Vulvar vestibulitis and interstitial cystitis: A disorder of uro-genital sinus-derived epithelium? *Obstetrics and Gynecology, 81,* 860-862.

Fordney, D.S. (1978). Dyspareunia and vaginismus. *Clinical Obstetrician Gynecology, 21,* 205-221.

Frank, R.T. (1948). Dyspareunia: A problem for the general practitioner. *Journal of the American Medical Association, 136,* 361-365.

Friedrich, E.G. (1987). Vulvar vestibulitis syndrome. *Journal of Reproductive Medicine, 32,* 110-114.

Gillenwater, J. & Wein, A. (1988) Summary of the National Institutes of Arthritis, Diabetes, Digestive and Kidney Disease workshop on Interstitial Cystitis, National Institutes of Health,

Bethesda, Maryland, August 28-29. *Journal of Urology, 140,* 203-206.

Gillespie, L. (1986). *You don't have to live with cystitis.* New York: Rawson Associates.

Goetsch, M.F. (1999). Post-partum dyspareunia: An unexplained problem. *Journal of Reproductive Medicine, 44,* 963-968.

Glatt, A.E., Zinner, S.H. & McCormack, W.M. (1990). *The prevalence of dyspareunia. Obstetrician and Gynecology, 75,* 433-536.

Gottleb, A. (1995) Post traumatic stress disorder and vulvar pain. *The Vulvar Pain Newsletter.* Graham, N.C.: Vulvar Pain Foundation, Fall.

Halvorsen, J.G. & Metz, M.E. (1992). Sexual dysfunction, part 1: Classification, etiology, and pathogenesis. *Journal of American Board Family Practitioner, 5,* 51-61.

Heim, L. (2001). Evaluation and differential diagnosis of dyspareunia. *American Family Physician, 63,* 1535-1544.

Held, P., Hanno, P., Wein, A., Pauly, M., & Cahn, M. (1990). Epidemiology of interstitial cystitis: 2. In P. Hanno, D. Staskin, R. Karne & A.Wein (Eds), *Interstitial Cystitis,* pp.29-48. New York: Springer-Verlag.

Herman, S. (1989). *Interstitial cystitis: Impact on female sexual function.* Paper presented at the meeting of the Society for the Scientific Study of Sexuality, Toronto, Canada.

Holm-Bentzen, M. & Lose, G. (1987). Pathology and pathogenesis of interstitial cystitis. *Urology Supplement, 29,* 8-13.

Huffman, J.W. (1976). Office gynecology: Relieving dyspareunia. *Post-Graduate Medicine, 59,* 223-226.

Kaplan, H. (1974). *The New Sex Therapy*. New York: Brummer Mazel.

Kessler, J. (1988). When the diagnosis is vaginismus: Fighting Misconceptions. *Women & Therapy, 7(2-3)*, 175-186.

Jamieson, D.J. & Steege, J.F. (1996). The prevalence of dysmenorrhea, dyspareunia, pelvic pain, and irritable bowel syndrome in primary care practices. *Obstetrician and Gynecology, 87*, 55-58.

Laumann, E., Paik, A. & Rosen, R.C. (1999). Sexual dysfunctions in the United States: Prevalence and predictors. *Journal of the American Medical Association, 281*, 537-544

Lazarus, A. (1980). Psychological treatment of dyspareunia. In Leblum, S.R. & Pervin, L.A. (1980) *Principles and practices of sex therapy*. New York: Guilford.

Leiblum, S. & Rosen, R. (2000). *Principles and Practice of Sex Therapy*. New York: Guilford Press.

Mann, M.S., Kaufman, R.H., Brown, D. & Adam, E. (1992). *Obstetrician and Gynecology, 79*, 122-125.

Marinoff, S.C. & Turner, M.L. (1991) Vulvar vestibulitis syndrome: an overview. American *Journal of Obstetrician and Gynecology, 165*, 1228-1232.

Masters, W. & Johnson, V. (1970). *Human Sexual inadequacy*. Boston: Little Brown.

McCormick, N. & Vinson, R. (1988). Sexual difficulties experiences by women with interstitial cystitis. *Women & Therapy, 7*, 109-119.

McCormick, N. (1995). Undesirable sexual side effects of medications. *ICA Update, 10(2)*, 5-6.

McKay, M. (1989). Vulvodynia: A multifactorial clinical problem. *Archives of Dermatology, 125*, 256-262.

McKay, M. (1991). Vulvitis and vulvovaginitis: Cutaneous consideration. *American Journal of Obstetricians and Gynecology, 165*, 1176-1182.

McKay, M. (1993). Dysesthetic ("essential") vulvodynia. Treatment with amitriptyline. *Journal of Reproductive Medicine, 38,* 9-13.

Meana, M., & Binik, Y.M (1994). Painful coitus: a review of female dyspareunia. *Journal of Nervous and Mental Disorders, 182,* 264-272.

Meana, M., Binik, Y.M., & Khalife, S. (1997). Bio-psychosocial profile of women with dyspareunia. *Obstetrician and Gynecology, 90,* 583-589.

Meana, M., Binik, Y.M., Khalife, S. & Cohen, D. (1997). Dyspareunia: sexual dysfunction or pain syndrome? *Journal of Nervous and Mental Disorders, 185*, 561-569.

Meana, M., Binik, Y.M., Khalife, S. & Cohen, D. (1998). Affect and marital adjustment in women's rating of dyspareunia pain. *Canadian Journal of Psychiatry, 43,* 381-385.

Paavonen, J. (1995). Diagnosis and treatment of vulvodynia. *Annuals of Medicine, 27*, 175-181.

Sandberg, G. & Quevillon, R.P. (1987). Dyspareunia: An integrated approach to assessment and diagnosis. *Journal of Family Practice, 24*, 66-69.

Sarazin, S.K. & Seymour, S.F. (1991). Causes and treatment options for women with dyspareunia. *Nurse Practitioner, 16*, 30-41.

Schellen, T. (1983). Dyspareunia: An increasing symptom in gynecology. *International Journal of Fertility, 28,* 116-118.

Spano, L. & Lamont (1975). Dyspareunia: A symptom of female sexual dysfunction. *Canadian Nursing, 71,* 22-25.

Spector, I.P. & Carey, M.P. (1990). Incidence and prevalence of the sexual dysfunctions: A critical review of the empirical literature. *Archives of Sexual Behavior, 19,* 389-408.

Steege, J.F. & Ling, F.W. (1993). Dyspareunia: A special type of chronic pelvic pain. *Obstetrician and Gynecology Clinics in North America, 20,* 779-793.

Turner, M.L. & Marinoff, S.C. (1988). Association of human papillomavirus with vulvodynia and the vulvar vestibulitis syndrome. *Journal of Reproductive Medicine, 33,* 533-537.

Walker, E., Katon, W., Harrop-Griffiths, J., Holm, L., Russo, J., Hickoc, L.R. (1988). Relationship of chronic pelvic pain to psychiatric diagnoses and childhood sexual abuse. *American Journal of Psychiatry, 145,* 75-80.

Webster, D. (1993). Sex and IC: Explaining the pain and planning self-care. *Urologic Nursing, 13,* 4-11.

Webster, D. (1996). Sex, Lies, and Stereotypes: Women and Interstitial Cystitis. *Journal of Sex Research, 33,* 197-203.

Webster, D. & Brennan, T. (1995). Use and effectiveness of sexual self-care strategies for interstitial cystitis. *Urologic Nursing, 15 (1),* 14-22.

Chapter 10

Althof, S.E. (1995). Pharmacologic treatment of rapid ejaculation. *Psychiatric Clinics of North American, 18,* 85-94.

Aizenberg, D., Zemishlany, Z., Hermesh, H., Karp, L. & Weizman, A. (1991). Painful ejaculation associated with antidepressants in four patients. *Journal of Clinical Psychiatry, 52*, 461-461.

American Psychiatric Association (1994). *Diagnostic and Statistical manual of Mental Disorders, 4th ed*, APA, Washington, DC.

Assalian, P. (1991, Nov.) *Premature ejaculation: Is it really psychogenic?* Paper presented at the annual meeting of the Society for the scientific Study of Sexuality, New Orleans, LA.

Beaumont, g. (1973). Sexual side-effects of clomipramine. *Journal of International Medical Research,1*, 469.

Colpi, G.M., Fanciullacci, F., Beretta, G., Negri, L., & Zanollo, A. (1986). Evoked sacral potentials in subjects with true premature ejaculation. *Andrologia, 18*, 583-586.

Cooper, R. & Magnus, R. (1984). A clinical trial of the beta blocker propranolol in premature ejaculation. *Journal of Psychosomatic Research, 28*, 331-336.

Darling, C.A., Davidson, J.K., & Cox, R.P. (1991). Females sexual response and the timing of partner orgasm. *Journal of Sex and Marital Therapy, 17*, 3-21.

DeAmicis, L.A., Goldberg, D.C., LoPiccolo, J. Friedman, J., & Davies, L. (1985). Clinical follow-up of couples treated for sexual dysfunction. *Archives of Sexual Behavior, 14*, 467-489.

Diakow, C. (1974). Male-female interactions and the organization of mammalian mating patterns. *Advances in the study of behavior, 5*, 227-268.

Ehrentheil, O/F. (1974). A case of premature ejaculation in Greek mythology. *Journal of Sex Research, 10*, 128-131.

Ellis, H. (1936). *Studies in the Psychology of Sex.* Random House: New York.

Foote, N. (1954). Sex as play. *Social Problems, 1,* 159-163.

Gebhard, P. H. (1966). Factors in marital orgasm. *Journal of Social Issues, 22,* 88-95.

Gospodinoff, P.H. (1989). Premature ejaculation: Clinical subgroups and etiology. *Journal of Sex and Martial Therapy, 15,* 130-134.

Grenier, G. & Byers, S. (1993). Controlling ejaculation: Reality or pipe dream. In Byers, E.S., *Testing common Assumptions about Human Sexuality.* Symposium presented at the meeting of the Canadian Psychological Association, Montreal.

Grenier, G. & Byers, S. (1995). Rapid ejaculation: A review of conceptual, etiological, and treatment issues. *Archives of Sexual Behavior, 24,* 447-472.

Hawton, K & Catalan, J. (1986). Prognostic factors in sex therapy. *Behavior Research and Therapy, 24,* 377-385.

Hong, L.K. (1984). Survival of the fastest: On the origin of premature ejaculation. *Journal of Sex Research, 20,* 109-122.

Kaplan, H. S. (1974). *The New Sex Therapy.* Brunner/Mazel: New York.

Kilmann, P.R. & Auerbach, R. (1979). Treatment of premature ejaculation and psychogenic impotence: A critical review of the literature. *Archives of Sexual Behavior, 8,* 81-100.

Kilmann, P.R., Boland, J.P., Noton, S.P., Davidson, E., & Caid, C. (1986). Perspectives of sex therapy outcome: A survey of AASECT providers. *Journal of Sex and Marital Therapy, 12,* 116-138.

Kinsey, A.C ..., Pomeroy, W.B. & Martin, C.E. (1948). *Sexual behavior in the human male.* W.B. Saunders: Philadelphia.

Kockott, G., Feil, W. Ferstl, R., Aldenhoff, J., & Besinger, U. (1980). Psycho-physiological aspects of male sexual inadequacy: Results of an experimental study. *Archives of Sexual Behavior, 9,* 477-493.

Lancaster, J.B. (1979). Sex and gender in evolutionary perspectives. In H.A. Katchdourian (Ed.) *Human Sexuality: A comparative and developmental perspective,* pp. 51-80. Berkeley: University of California Press.

Levine, S. B. (1992). *Sexual Life: A Clinician's Guide.* Plenum Press: New York.

LoPiccolo, J. (1978). Direct treatment of sexual dysfunction in the couple. In Money, J. & Mesaph, H. (eds.), *Handbook of Sexology: Vol. 5., Selected syndromes and therapy.* Elsevier: New York, pp. 1227-1244.

Masters, W. & Johnson, V. (1970). *Human Sexual Inadequacy.* Little and Brown: Boston.

Montiero, W., Noshirvani, H. Marks, I., & Lelliott, P. (1987) Anorgasmia from clomipramine in obsessive-compulsive disorder. A controlled trial. *British Journal of Psychiatry, 151,* 107-112.

Reading, A. & Wiest, W. (1984). An analysis of self-reported sexual behavior in a sample of normal males. *Archives of Sexual behavior, 13,* 69-83.

Rowland, D.L., Greenleaf, W., Mas., M., Myers, L., & Davidson, J. M. (1989). Penile and finger sensory thresholds in young, aging, and diabetic males. *Archive of Sexual Behavior, 18,* 1-12.

Ruff, G.A. & St. Lawrence, J. S. (1985). Premature ejaculation: Past research progress, future direction. *Clinical Psychological Review,* 5, 627-639.

Rust, J., Golombok, S., & Collier, J. (1988). Marital problems and sexual dysfunction: How are they related? *British Journal of Psychiatry, 152,* 629-631.

Schover, L. R., Friedman, J.M., Weiler, S.J., Heiman, J.R. & Lopiccolo, J. (1982). Multi-axial problem-oriented system for sexual dysfunction. *Archives of General Psychiatry, 39,* 614-619.

Segraves, R.T. (1989). Effects of psychotropic drugs on human erection and ejaculation. *Archives of General Psychiatry, 46,* 275-284.

Segraves, R. T., saran, A., Segraves, K. & Maguire, E. (1992). *Clomipramine vs. placebo in the treatment of premature ejaculation.* Paper presented at the meeting of the International Academy of Sex Research, Prague, Czechoslovakia.

Semans, J. H. (1956). Premature ejaculation: A new approach. *Southern Medical Journal, 49,* 353-358.

Shilon, M., Paz, G.F., & Homonnai, Z. T. (1984). The use of phenoxybenzamine treatment in premature ejaculation. *Fertility and Sterility, 42,* 659-661.

Spector, I.P. & Carey, M.P. (1990). Incidence and prevalence of the sexual dysfunction: A critical review of the empirical literature. *Archives of Sexual Behavior, 19,* 389-408.

Spiess, W.F., Geer, J.H., & O'Donohue, W.T. (1984). Premature ejaculation: Investigation of factors in ejaculatory latency. *Journal of Abnormal Psychology, 93,* 242-245.

Strassberg, D.S., Kelly, M.P., Carroll, C., & Kircher, J.C. (1987). The psychophysiological nature of premature ejaculation. *Archives of Sexual Behavior, 16,* 327-336.

Strassberg, d. S., Mahoney, J.M., Schaugaard, M., & Hale, V.E. (1990). The role of anxiety in premature ejaculation: A psychophysiological model. *Archives of Sexual Behavior, 19,* 251—258.

Williams, W. (1984). Secondary premature ejaculation. *Australian Journal of Psychiatry, 18,* 333-340.

Wolpe, J. (1982). *The practice of behavior therapy, 3ʳᵈ ed.* Pergamon: Toronto.

Zilbergeld, B. (1987). *Male Sexuality.* Bantam: Toronto.

Chapter 11

Clarke, A.E., Ruble, D.N. (1978). Young adolescents' behavior concerning menstruation. *Child Development, 49,* 231-234.

Clement, V., Schmidt, G., Kruse, M. (1984). Change in sexual differences in sexual behavior: A replication of a study on West German students (1966-1981). *Archives of Sexual Behavior, 13,* 99-120.

Clifford, R. (1987). Development of Masturbation in college women. *Archives of Sexual Behavior, 7,* 573-599.

Daly, M. (1978). *Gyn/Ecology—The metaethics of radical feminism.* Boston: Beacon Press.

Darling, C.A., Davidson, J.K. (1966). Coitally active university students: Sexual behavior, concerns and challenges. *Adolescence, 21,* 403-419.

deBruijn, G. (1982). From masturbation to orgasm with a partner: How some women bridge the gap—and why others don't. *Journal of Sex and Marital Therapy, 8,* 151-167.

Doyle, J.A. (1983). *The Male Experience.* Dubuque, IA: William C. Brown.

Fisher, S. (1973). *The Female Orgasm: Psychology, Physiology, Fantasy.* New York: Basic Books, Inc.

Gagnon, W. (1981). *Review of Medical Physiology.* Los Altos, California: Lange Medical Publications.

—(1988). Attitudes and responses of parent to pre-adolescent masturbation. *Archives of Sexual Behavior, 14,* 451-466.

Giorgis, B. (1981). *Female circumcision in Africa.* United Nations Economic Commission for Africa.

Hite, S. (1976). *The Hite report: A nationwide study of female sexuality.* New York: Dell Publishing.

Kinsey, A.C., Pomeroy, W.B., Martin, C., Gebhard, P. (1953). *Sexual behavior in the Human Female.* Philadelphia: W.B. Saunders.

Logan, D. (1980). The menarche experience in twenty-three foreign countries. *Adolescence, 15,* 247-256.

Masters, W. Johnson, V. (1966). *Human sexual response.* Boston: Little & Brown.

Polonko, K, A. (1990). Patriarchal scripts and frequency of orgasm during coitus. (unpublished)

Reinish, J.M. (1990). *The Kinsey Institutes new report on sex.* New York: St. Martin's Press.

Reynolds, B. (1994). The move to outlaw female genital mutilation. *Ms., July/August, 92-93.*

Roberts, E.J., Kline, D., Gagnon, J. (1978). *Family life and sexual learning.* Cambridge Mass. Project of human sexual development, Popular Education.

Shaw, E. (1985). Female circumcision. *American journal of nursing,* June, 684-687.

Shotly, M.J., Ephross, P.H., Plaut, S.M., Fischman, S.H., Charnas, J.F., Cody, C.A ... (1984). Female orgasmic experience: A subjective study. *Archives of Sexual Behavior, 13,* 155-163.

Slack, A.T. (1988). Female circumcision: A critical appraisal. *Human Rights Quarterly, 10,* 437-486.

Udry, J.R., Talbert, L.M., Morris, N.M. (1986). Biological foundations for adolescent female sexuality. *Demography, 2,* 217-227.

Wilson, W.C. (1975). The distribution of selected sexual attitudes and behaviors among the adult population of the United States. *Journal of Sex Research, 11,* 46-64.

Chapter 12

Brabham, E.G. & Villaume, S.K. (2003). Scientifically Based Reading Research—A Call for an Expanded View. *Reading Teacher, 56,* 698-701.

Martin, K. & Bearden, D. (1998). Listserv Learning. *Learning and Leading with Technology,* 26, 39-41.

Overbaugh, R. (1998). Large-Group E-mail Communication: Management Nightmare and the Listserv Solution. *Clearing house, 71,* 355-358.

Robinson, K. (1996). People Talking to People: Making the most of Internet Discussion Groups. *Online, 20*, 26-30,32.

Villaume, S.K. & Brabham, E.G. (2002). Comprehension Instruction: Beyond Strategies. *Reading Teacher, 55*, 672-675.

Chapter 13

Bartell, G. (1970). Group sex among the mid-Americans. *Journal of Sexual Research, 6*, 113-130.

Bartell, G. (1971). *Group Sex.* New York: Wyden.

Bezilla, R.E. (1993). *Religion in America*, Princeton Religion Research Center, Princeton, New Jersey.

Denfeld, D. (1974). Dropouts from swinging. The family Coordinator, 23, 45-49.

Felton, J. (1984). A Psychoanalytic Perspective on Sexually Open relations. *Psychoanalytic Review, 71*, 279-295.

Flanigan, W.H. & Zingale,N.H. (1991). *Political Behavior of the American electorate* (7th Ed.), CQ Press, Washington, DC.

Freud, S. (1908). Civilized Sexuality and Modern Nervous Illness. *Standard Edition, 9*. London: Hogarth, 1959.

Freud, S. (1912). On the Universal tendency to debasement in the Sphere of Love. *Standard Edition, 2*. London: Hogarth, 1959.

Gallup, G. & Castelli, J. (1989). *The People's religion: American faith in the 90's.* Macmillian: New York.

Gediman, H. (1975). Romanticism, Narcissism, and Creativity. *Journal of American Psychoanalysis Association, 23*.

Gilmartin, B. G. (1975). The swingers next door. *Psychology Today, 8,* 54-58.

Henshel, A.M. (1973). Swinging: A study of decision making in marriage. *American Journal of Sociology, 4,* 885-891.

Jenks, R. (1985a). A comparative study of swinger and non-swinger: Attitudes and beliefs. Lifestyles: *Journal of Changing Patterns, 7,* 5-20.

Jenks, R. (1985b). Swinging: A replication and test of a theory. *Journal of Sex Research, 21,* 199-205.

Jenks, R. (1986). *A further analysis of swinging.* Unpublished manuscript.

Knapp, J.J. & Whitehurst, R.N. (1977). Sexually open marriages and relationships: Issues and prospects. In R.W. Libby & R.N. Whitehurst (Eds.) *Marriage and alternatives: Exploring intimate relations, pp. 147-160.* Glenview, Il: Scott, Foresman.

Levitt, E. E. (1988) Alternative life styles and marital satisfaction: A brief report. *Annals of Sex Research, 1,* 455-461.

O'Neill, N. (1973). Interview by the editors. *Single,* August.

O'Neill, N. (1977). *The Marriage premise.* New York: M. Evans.

O'Neill, N. & O'Neill, G. (1972). Open Marriage: A new lifestyle for couples. New York: M. Evans.

O'Neill, N. & O'Neill, G. (1974). Open Marriage: The conceptual framework. In Smith, J.R & Smith,L.G. (eds.), *Beyond Monogamy: Recent studies on Sexual Alternatives in Marriage,* Johns Hopkins Press: Baltimore.

Rubin, A. M. & Adams, J. R. (1986). Outcomes of Sexually Open Marriages. The *Journal of Sex Research, 22*, 311-319.

Safilios-Rothschild, Constantina (1970). The study of family power structure: A review 1960-1969. *Journal of Marriage and the Family, 32*, 539-552.

Stinnett, N. & Birdsong, C.W. (1978). *The Family and Alternate Lifestyles*. Nelson-Hall: Chicago.

Varni, C.A. (1974). An exploratory study of spouse swapping. In Smith, J.R & Smith,L.G. (eds.), Beyond Monogamy: Recent studies on Sexual Alternatives in Marriage, Johns Hopkins Press: Baltimore.

978-0-595-45985-8
0-595-45985-4

www.ingramcontent.com/pod-product-compliance
Lightning Source LLC
Chambersburg PA
CBHW030259290526
45785CB00001B/140